BIOETHICS AND THE
CATHOLIC MORAL TRADITION

BIOETHICS
and the Catholic Moral Tradition

Rev. Dr Pádraig Corkery

VERITAS

Published 2010 by
Veritas Publications
7–8 Lower Abbey Street
Dublin 1
Ireland
publications@veritas.ie
www.veritas.ie

ISBN 978-1-84730-245-8

Copyright © Pádraig Corkery, 2010

10 9 8 7 6 5 4 3 2 1

The material in this publication is protected by copyright law. Except as may be permitted by law, no part of the material may be reproduced (including by storage in a retrieval system) or transmitted in any form or by any means, adapted, rented or lent without the written permission of the copyright owners. Applications for permissions should be addressed to the publisher.

A catalogue record for this book is available from the British Library.

Cover designed by Tanya M. Ross
Typesetting by Barbara Croatto
Printed in Ireland by Hudson Killeen, Dublin

Veritas books are printed on paper made from the wood pulp of managed forests. For every tree felled, at least one tree is planted, thereby renewing natural resources.

Contents

Introduction   7

Section One
Catholic Moral Teaching: The Sources

1. A Catholic Christian Approach to Bioethics   11

Section Two
The Content of Catholic Moral Teaching

2. Assisted Human Reproduction   41
3. Embryonic Stem Cell Research   59
4. Ethical Issues at the End of Life   79
5. The Administration of Nutrition and Hydration to Persons in a Permanent Vegetative State (PVS)   92

Section Three
Catholic Moral Teaching and the Individual

6. The Nature and Role of Personal Conscience   111

Section Four
Catholic Moral Teaching and Society

7. Morality and the Civil Law   129

Introduction

OVER THE PAST FEW DECADES, DEVELOPMENTS IN medicine and medical science have fascinated individuals and societies across the globe. People have been held spellbound by the many new developments that have contributed richly to the health, quality of life and longevity of humankind. At the same time, questions about the rightness or the ethical nature of some of these developments in medical science have been the source of debate and sharp disagreement in many societies.

The purpose of this brief introduction to bioethics is to examine some of the more controversial of these developments and practices from the perspective of the Catholic moral tradition. To facilitate the process of reflection, the book is broken into four uneven sections, each of which responds to a particular question. The first section, comprising chapter one, responds to questions about the *sources or roots* of moral teaching in the Catholic moral tradition. What are the sources used by the Catholic Church in reflecting on, and formulating a response to, contemporary moral issues? The second section, containing four chapters, responds to questions about the *content* of Catholic moral teaching. What exactly are the conclusions of the Catholic moral tradition on, for example, euthanasia or embryonic stem cell research? The penultimate section, containing chapter six, engages with questions concerning the relationship between the *individual* and Church teaching. In particular, it examines the nature, formation and role of *personal conscience*. The final section and chapter responds to concerns about the relationship between Church teaching and society. What relevance have the conclusions of the Catholic moral tradition for the ethos of *society* and, in particular, the content of the civil law?

This book is intended for a general audience, rather than a specialised academic one. It does not engage, therefore, with the debate within Catholic moral theology on certain aspects and nuances of Catholic moral teaching. Neither does it attempt to engage with the ongoing debates between professional ethicists and academics across the globe. Its goal is more modest and limited: to outline the *what* and the *why* of Catholic teaching in the area of bioethics. After studying this text, students of theology, parish-based adult education groups and individual searchers will, I hope, have a clear grasp of the approach and conclusions of the Catholic moral tradition to some of today's bioethical issues. Each chapter concludes with a series of questions and a short reading list that may facilitate more in-depth study and discussion.

Section One

Catholic Moral Teaching: The Sources

1 A Catholic Christian Approach to Bioethics

THE QUESTION OF WHETHER THERE IS A CATHOLIC Christian bioethic or a distinctive Christian approach to bioethics is an important one that needs to be teased out at the very beginning of this project. How does the Christian and, in particular, the Catholic tradition evaluate actions and attitudes in the domain of healthcare that are often complex? What are the sources of wisdom employed by Christian teachers and theologians to guide their decisions on issues as diverse as embryonic stem cell research and behaviour modification?

The Catholic tradition employs three sources of wisdom that enable it to reach moral conclusions on specific issues. These fonts of wisdom are the Christian Scriptures, the ongoing living tradition of a believing community and, finally, the natural law tradition. These can be clearly seen in the following quotation from *Evangelium vitae*, which identifies the sources used by the Church when formulating its opposition to euthanasia:

> This doctrine is based upon the natural law and upon the written word of God, is transmitted by the Church's Tradition and taught by the ordinary and universal Magisterium.[1]

At the outset of this introduction to bioethics from the Catholic tradition, it is important to identify, as sharply as possible, what each of these sources of wisdom have to offer moral reflection in the complex and dynamic world of bioethics.

1. THE CHRISTIAN SCRIPTURES

From the outset, we can say with certainty that the Christian Scriptures do not give us clear and unambiguous answers to many of the questions in contemporary healthcare. Nor should we expect them to. The primary purpose of Scripture is *revelation*: to reveal to us God and God's interventions in human history. In the course of telling us about God, Scripture does, of course, tell us something about morality – but that is not its primary purpose. It was not, therefore, written as a rulebook that sets out clear and unambiguous answers to complicated questions. The book of the Christian Scriptures was also written, over a long period of time, in very different contexts and cultures and, therefore, its horizons are very different to ours.

If Scripture is not a rulebook that provides us with immediate answers to contemporary questions, we are entitled to ask how it helps us in moral reflection. This question has been reflected on by the Magisterium and Catholic theologians over many years, but particularly since Vatican II. One of the most important renewals promoted by Vatican II was that of moral theology, the discipline of the Catholic theological tradition that reflects on the moral implications of human activity in light of the Christian message. In particular, the Council insisted that moral theology and moral reflection should be nourished and rooted in the Scriptures. Since then, Catholic theologians and the Magisterium have attempted to put Scripture at the heart of moral reflection.[2] Part of this ongoing journey is to tease out exactly how we can use the moral teachings of the Scriptures in our reflections on contemporary issues that have no resonance with the culture and issues of biblical times. A recent publication from the Pontifical Biblical Commission is a good example of a scholarly reflection on this subject, which sets out useful criteria to enable an engagement between Scripture and contemporary moral reflection.[3] In the course of this section we will engage with this text in some detail.

From the outset of our reflection, we can say that the Scriptures give us a unique framework or worldview from which we can approach the issues that confront us today. They provide us with a narrative or canvas that gives us a very particular stance on life. In a decisive manner, the Christian Scriptures give us a way of understanding ourselves, the world we inhabit and others. We all work out of a worldview that impacts decisively on what we see as important and informs our decision-making. The Christian worldview or stance on life can be reflected on under several headings.

God as the Loving Creator of the Universe we Inhabit
In the Christian self-understanding, the world we inhabit is a gift from a loving and personal God. Moreover, it is a world that is good with its own purpose and internal logic. It was given to humankind as a 'gift' to be used wisely and responsibly. This is a very different starting point from one that views creation as a result of random chance with no inbuilt purpose or goal. The important thing to note here is that this starting point or worldview does have an impact on how we evaluate our relationship with the created order. If God is the Creator, then, in the language of the Christian tradition, we are 'creatures' called to use wisely and responsibly the gifts we have been given. If we are 'creatures', then by implication we are not the Lord of creation. God alone is Lord.

A contemporary rendering of this insight argues that we are called to be 'responsible stewards' of the creation gifted to us. This self-understanding places obvious and immediate limits on human interventions in God's creation. We are not free to manipulate or interfere with creation in a random and haphazard way. Rather, our interventions must respect the nature and value of the 'gift' we have been entrusted with. This insight is central to the developing Catholic literature on ecology as a moral issue. In his recent encyclical, Pope Benedict XVI argued that creation contains a 'grammar' that explains its nature and purpose.[4] As responsible stewards we are called to respect and honour this 'grammar' in our engagements with creation.[5]

Created in 'God's Image'
The Christian worldview proposes a very particular view of the human person – a Christian anthropology.[6] In this understanding, the human person is created 'in the image of God'. There are several implications that flow from this assertion that have profound implications for how we engage with people and what we see as important in life. In the first place, the Christian tradition claims that *all* persons are created in the 'image of God', not just a select few or the virtuous. There is a radical equality among people that needs to be respected in our daily engagements with others and in our political and social structures. Sadly, both the Church and wider society were slow to honour this implication of Christian anthropology. Today, thankfully, the equality of persons is almost universally recognised in principle, but still needs to be honoured in practice in many different societies and structures.

Because we are created in the *'imago Dei'* we each have a dignity that is intrinsic to us. It flows from our very nature as sons and daughters created by God and in the 'likeness' of

God. Each one of us in some mysterious way reflects the life and love of our Creator. Biblical authors used human language and images, the only descriptive 'tools' available to them, to describe this awesome truth.[7] The important point here is that our dignity is *intrinsic* to us. It is not dependant on our health, wealth, achievements, sexual orientation or religious affiliation. This Christian claim is in direct opposition to some contemporary worldviews that would link human dignity to achievement, sexual orientation or health.

Secondly, our creation in 'God's image' reveals that there is a Godly or spiritual dimension to each person. Christian anthropology asserts that we come from God and go to God; God is our origin and destiny. This Godly or transcendent dimension needs to be acknowledged and nourished if we are to adequately engage with the person in society. This truth about the human person boldly proclaims that we are more than one-dimensional. We are an integrated totality of body and spirit. Consequently, in the words of the Gospel, we are not satisfied by bread alone. This aspect of Christian anthropology informs Christian reflections on the phenomenon of consumerism and some political philosophies that reduce the person to a one-dimensional existence. The Christian tradition, in contrast, claims that human fulfilment is to be found in *being* more rather than *having* more.[8]

Finally, the creation account in the Book of Genesis reveals that the need for relationships is a fundamental dimension of human existence. Human persons are social by nature, called into a web of relationships that enable the person to blossom and reach their potential. We are, in the Christian tradition, always understood as 'persons-in-community', called to relationships of mutuality, love and respect. This aspect of our nature has significant implications for the spheres of politics, economics and social policy that are well teased out in the growing corpus of Catholic social doctrine. The principles of the common good and solidarity, in particular, honour this dimension of human existence and its implications for the societies we inhabit and construct.[9]

To summarise, then, the understanding of the person as created in the '*imago Dei*' has decisive implications for our engagement with people and for what we see as important when we are involved in moral decision-making.

The Sin of Adam and Eve

An important dimension of Christian anthropology and of the Christian worldview is that humanity is sinful and finite. The biblical authors brilliantly describe this reality in their account of the sin of Adam and Eve in the Book of Genesis. Our first parents, motivated by the desire for power and tempted by Satan, disobeyed God by eating of the apple. The consequences of this action are told to us in *relational* terms. The relationships of respect and mutuality that existed up to that point were ruptured and replaced by relationships of domination and shame. Adam and Eve fought with each other while attempting to place the blame on the other. Their relationship of mutuality was replaced by one of domination.[10] Both were ashamed before God and tried to hide. The cosy relationship between the world of nature and humankind was replaced by a relationship of enmity and toil. Adam and Eve had to leave paradise and earn their bread by the sweat of their brow in a sometimes hostile environment.

This account of the human condition as sinful and prone to selfishness is part of the Christian worldview and self-understanding. It is part of the canvas or background against which Christians work and conduct their moral reflections. It gives a realistic picture of the human condition and alerts us to the danger of self-deception and self-preoccupation. In particular, it calls us to be alert to the sins of pride and selfishness and how those sins may impact on our behaviour and moral reflections.

The Person of Christ

In the Christian self-understanding, the person of Christ has a defining role. Christians understand themselves as a community formed in His name and are inspired to shape their lives around His example. Christians, of all denominations, see themselves as disciples of Christ called to witness to Him and the values of the Gospel in the world. Through their daily lives, they see themselves contributing to the transformation of the world and the building up of God's kingdom. For them the person and example of Christ are normative.[11] In the words of the Gospel, Christians are called to 'do likewise' and to be the 'salt of the earth and the light of the world'.

It is a central part of the Christian self-understanding that Christ came among us as a model of right relationships. His person, actions and attitudes show us how to live out our lives in keeping with our nature and dignity as sons and daughters of God. We believe that his behaviour is not only instructive, but normative for all who strive to live 'the good life'.

In the Gospels, Christ calls us to be a particular kind of person: kind, loving, forgiving, and so on. The character of the follower of Christ is beautifully unpacked in the many parables and stories recorded in the four Gospels. The Prodigal Son (Lk 15:11-31), the Good Samaritan (Lk 10:29-37), The Pharisee and the Tax Collector (Lk 18:9-14) and the Widow's Mite (Mk 12:41-44) all highlight different aspects of the disciple's character. The Beatitudes (Mt 5:1-12) express even more clearly the horizons out of which we are called to live our lives. We are invited to allow these stories to shape our imaginations and set our horizons so that we, too, will become forgiving, compassionate and loving people. Moral theology calls these elements of the Gospel 'formal norms' because they call and enable us to become a particular kind of person: a Christ-like person, who acts with justice, love and compassion.

But, you may ask, is there anything more concrete in the life of Christ and the Gospel narratives? The emphasis on love, compassion, interiority and service of others is, you might suggest, very vague and unhelpful. We need something more concrete and definite in order to engage with contemporary moral issues! There are, of course, moral teachings in the life of Christ and, indeed, in the Old Testament that are more focused and definite. The Ten Commandments and Christ's teaching on divorce spring immediately to mind. These are what moral theologians have called 'material or concrete norms'. Although these are helpful they are not unproblematic, as the treatment of the fifth commandment today and over the centuries has shown. There is need to distinguish between specific moral teachings that are universally binding and those that are culturally conditioned or case sensitive.

Resurrection Destiny

The final element of the worldview, or landscape, that Christians work out of is that of resurrection destiny. We believe that as Christ rose from the dead to new life, we, too, will share that destiny. This faith is prayerfully articulated in the Preface of the Mass for the Dead: 'Lord, for your faithful people life is changed not ended. When our earthly body lies in death we gain an everlasting dwelling place in heaven.'

The reality of Christian hope is an important element in the Christian worldview that has significant consequences for how we engage with suffering and death. Our moral reflections on, say, martyrdom or issues at the end of life, including euthanasia, are deeply shaped by faith in a resurrection to new life. Equally, the moral reflections of those who are without hope of resurrection, who view death as the final and defining reality, are shaped by that belief.

The Scriptures then provide the framework or context out of which Christians live their lives and engage in moral reflection. Belief in a loving creator God, in the person of Christ and in eternal life gives Christians a unique orientation in life. This orientation includes the identification of certain attitudes and actions as life-giving and moral, and others as contrary to morality. Questions still remain, however, as to the precise role the Scriptures play in moral reflection. Because the Scriptures contain many passages that are concerned with human behaviour and morality, we must have some criteria to enable us to determine those that are of abiding significance.

We can be clear, as stated earlier, about what the Scriptures cannot provide: clear and automatic answers to complex issues like those raised by recent developments in reproductive technologies. We cannot jump immediately from the pages of the Gospels or other scriptural texts and arrive at a conclusion about the morality of an issue that was beyond the wildest dreams of the scriptural authors. Our engaging with Christ and the Scriptures must be more patient, sophisticated and nuanced. Catholic biblical scholarship has, over recent decades, developed tools, like exegesis and hermeneutics, which enable us to engage with Scripture in ways that are respectful of its nature and limits and yet yield fruit for moral reflection. These tools help us to understand the context in which the Scriptures were written and the nature of the texts themselves. They also enable us to distinguish between moral teachings that are culturally conditioned and, therefore, not universally binding, and those that have an enduring validity. The Biblical Commission, in their recent publication, proposed two fundamental criteria and six specific criteria to help us draw moral insight from the Scriptures. The fundamental criteria it proposed, which we have encountered already, are the biblical understanding of the human person and the normative example of Christ. How we understand the human person has inevitable and significant consequences for moral reflection, as does the acceptance of Christ's life as normative for humanity. The six specific criteria proposed by the Biblical Commission, which I will now examine, are very helpful in enabling us to discern the relevance of the moral message of Scripture for today.[12] These criteria are: convergence, contrast, advance, the community dimension, finality and discernment. They were proposed by the Biblical Commission as essential tools in the ongoing conversation between Scripture and moral reflection. They enable us to identify the various kinds of moral norms in the Bible and their respective significance for moral reasoning. For that reason they are worthy of further elaboration.

Convergence[13]

The criterion of convergence recognises that there is frequently a convergence between the insights of the Bible and the insights of surrounding societies on morality. The Commission fleshed out this claim by citing numerous examples. Accounts of the creation of the world by a personal divinity, for example, and the origin of sin and evil contained in Genesis are also to be found in the accounts and myths found in other cultures. It is also true that the laws of the Old Testament (for example, Ex 20-23; Deut 12-26) also belong to the great legislative tradition of the ancient East like, for example, the code of Hammurabi.

Justice, and especially the protection of the weak, was the foundation of many societies in Near Eastern culture.[14] The Wisdom of the Bible shows a close resemblance also to 'the wisdom of Amenemope and Ptah-Hotep, especially on matters dealing with the protection of the weak and the vulnerable (cf Prov 22:17-24)'.[15] Finally, Paul acknowledges and appreciates the natural law in Romans 2:14-15 and integrates into his teaching themes that were very familiar to contemporary philosophers and teachers of morality. The best example, according to the Commission, occurs in Romans 7:16-24. This text deals with the enslavement of human beings to their habits and passions and their lack of true freedom. It was taken from Euripides' *Medea* and has parallels in Ovid (*Metamorphoses* 7:20-21) and Epictetus (*Dissertations* 2:17-19). Though it notes that many of Paul's 'stances and exhortations are close to those of the Stoics',[16] the text identifies Paul's originality with, among other things, his understanding of the role of the Spirit.

In terms of its relevance for today, the principle of convergence reminds us that Christians can join with others in looking for solutions to contemporary ethical issues. Our shared humanity and the natural law tradition provides the basis for dialogue and agreement among Christians and others. The principle is also a reminder that a Scripture-based morality is always reasonable and, therefore, accessible to people of good will everywhere.

Contrast[17]

The principle of contrast reminds us that the Bible is unambiguously opposed to certain norms and customs followed by some societies and individuals. This is clearly evident in the writings of the prophets and in the New Testament writings. The Commission developed the principle of contrast under the general rubric of idolatry or infidelity to God as Lord of all. The principle is clearly seen in the struggle of the prophets against idolatry[18] among the people of Israel. The prophets Hosea, Amos and Jeremiah, as well as others, rallied against the cult of Baal and the cult of home-made divinities (Hos 4:7-14, 10:1-2, 13:1-3; Amos 2:4-8; Jer 7:1-15). Enforced pagan worship is confronted and condemned in First and Second Maccabees and the Book of Wisdom.[19] Paul in his time voiced his opposition to pagan worship[20] and confronted the paganism of the Roman Empire in Acts 19:24-41. Finally, in the Book of Revelation we witness the confrontation between the kingdom of God and the anti-kingdom of Satan.[21]

The relevance and implication of this principle for today is that it mandates believers to confront attitudes and actions that are in opposition to God's ways and sovereignty. Modern forms of idolatry 'appear as self-idolatry, be it of individuals, social classes or states'.[22] When human freedom is elevated to a supreme value and when systems of thought or philosophy exclude any transcendent value they become idolatrous. For this reason the Christian tradition is rightly critical of and opposed to consumerism, materialism and hedonism. The principle of contrast, in short, motivates and enables believers to confront systems, attitudes and actions that usurp or deny God's place in our lives and world.

Advance[23]

The third principle, advance, highlights an important fact about biblical morality that has implications for how we engage with scriptural texts in moral argument. The content of the principle is that biblical morality, like revelation itself, progressed and developed in a gradual way. This development of biblical morality reached its peak in the coming of Christ, who confirmed and deepened the teaching of Moses and the prophets. Consequently, we must decipher the moral message of the Old Testament definitively in light of the New Testament. This principle alerts us to the danger of using biblical texts in isolation, as 'stand alone' texts, rather than interpreting and understanding them in light of the ethos of Christ's life and teaching.

The Commission's text took three examples of moral teaching to elucidate the principle of advance in biblical morality. The first example is that of conflict with one's neighbour. In biblical morality there is a gradual development in how such conflict is handled. There is an advance from excessive vengeance (Gen 4:23-24) to equality of retaliation (Ex 21:23-24) until, finally, the chain of retribution is overcome (Mt 5:38-42). Jesus goes beyond the earlier morality, found also in the law codes of other ancient oriental peoples, and introduces a radically new approach: 'But I say to you. Do not resist the evildoer. But if anyone strikes you on the right cheek …' (Mt 5:38-42).

The second example of advance concerns marriage.[24] In Matthew 5:31-32 and 19:8, Jesus brings to completion the gradual development of biblical teaching on the nature of marriage. In the Old Testament we find both polygamy (Gen 4:19, 29:21-30; 1 Sam 1:2, 25:43) and divorce (Deut 24:1-4). Jesus rejects these practices and roots his teaching in the original will of God the Creator. This teaching is carried on by Paul and the early Church (1 Cor 7:10-11).

The nature of divine worship is the third example of advance elaborated on in the Commission's text.[25] In Matthew 6:1-18, Jesus engaged with three important expressions of divine worship: almsgiving, prayer and fasting. He is critical, not of the practices themselves, but of the intention or attitude that often motivated these actions. The goal of these actions, he reminded his listeners, was to worship God and not to acquire praise from others or to become preoccupied with rubrics. Through Christ and the new covenant, a new kind of worship, which sets aside the old cultic system, is possible. This theme is well developed in the letter to the Hebrews 8:1–9:28, where the author underlines the superiority of the sacrifice of Christ and of the new covenant.

The implications of these three advances for those who embrace the Christian vision are, in the eyes of the Commission, 'an unlimited willingness to forgive, unconditional loyalty to one's chosen partner, and a spiritual and interior worship of God that leads on to a solid commitment to transformation of the world.'[26]

The Community Dimension[27]

The fourth specific criterion proposed by the Commission, in order to facilitate a dialogue between Scripture and moral reflection, is the community dimension of our existence and of morality. Throughout the Bible, the essential community dimension of morality is emphasised and rooted in the nature of the human person and God. In the Biblical perspective, the human person is not perceived as an isolated and autonomous individual, but as a member of a community. The implications of this are highlighted both in the Old Testament and the New Testament where morality is presented in a communitarian context. Paul and the other New Testament writers insist that the members of the new Christian community are 'bound to render true worship of God, to take care of others, to form a community of love and friendship, to share earthly goods so that no one is in need and to continue the mission of healing and reconciliation.'[28]

The text of the Commission highlights three implications of this community dimension of existence and morality. Within the community,[29] we are called to look after the weaker members of society, such as the classic trio in the Old

Testament: 'the widow, the orphan, and the foreigner' (Deut 16:11-12, 26:11-12). The New Testament uses the language of 'love your neighbour as yourself' (Mt 22:37-40) and the 'golden rule' in Matthew 7:12: 'Do to others as you would have them do to you'. Those on the margins of the community[30] must also be embraced and cared for. The Old Testament highlighted the need to include and love the alien (Lev 19:34), while Jesus' mission is presented as full of solicitude for the 'lost sheep'. The proclamation of the Gospel is characterised as 'good news for the poor' and is inclusive of sinners and others on the margins of society. Finally, biblical morality extends to the care of those outside the community.[31] The behaviour of Jesus in welcoming gentiles, including the Canaanite woman in Matthew 15:21-28 and the centurion in Luke 7:1-10, sets the standard for individuals and communities gathered in His name.

The criterion of community has obvious implications for the Christian family in today's world. It motivates the building of societies that are inclusive, caring and just. It stands as a powerful critique of individualism and indifference. Catholic social teaching has energetically embraced this biblical criterion in its ongoing task of critiquing the political, social and economic realities of the day. The principles of Catholic social teaching, especially those of the common good and the virtue of solidarity, bear witness to the centrality of this biblical criterion.

Finality[32]

The penultimate criterion proposed is that of finality. This is our Christian hope in a future life with God founded on Christ's resurrection. This hope gives believers a unique starting point for moral reflection and motivates and enables lifestyles that are in conformity with God's will. This hope of believers only gradually appeared in the Old Testament writings and is first seen clearly in the Maccabean period (2 Macc 7:9-36).[33] This hope is confirmed in the exchanges between Jesus and the Sadducees (Mk 12:18-29), in his preaching about the kingdom of heaven (Mt 7:21) and, definitively, in his resurrection. Paul, and the other New Testament writers, further developed the theme of resurrection and its link to the moral quality of our present life (1 Cor 15; Rom 14:10-12). Those who follow faithfully the example of Jesus will share a 'blessed life with the risen Christ'.[34]

The criterion of finality gives believers a particular stance on the present and the future. On the one hand, it makes us aware of the passing and limited nature of the present and, on the other hand, it directs us towards a future that is eternal. Such a stance leads to an engagement with the present, rather than an indifference, that strives with a lively hope to transform reality in light of the kingdom and its values. Such engagement is rooted in a confidence that ultimately God's kingdom will be established: life will prevail over death, light will prevail over darkness and goodness will prevail over evil.

Discernment[35]

The Commission in their study insisted that we cannot 'attribute equal value to all the examples of morality presented by Scripture'.[36] Therefore, prudence is needed to distinguish fundamental requirements, which have an obligatory universal value, from simple counsels and from precepts linked to a particular stage of spiritual development. Scripture itself, according to the Commission, provides us with three criteria that enable us to discern clearly in order to make sound decisions. These criteria are literary discernment, spiritual discernment on the level of the community and spiritual discernment on the personal level. *Literary discernment* obliges us, when looking at a particular narrative of the Bible, to take into account its literary context and to pay attention to literary genres and forms, since these often qualify the weight of an ethical discourse. When examining various norms proposed in the Bible, 'special attention must be paid to those supported by a theological foundation or justification'.[37] These criteria help us to distinguish rulings linked to a particular culture from those of trans-cultural value. It is also imperative to take into account the cultural background of a particular biblical norm when trying to discern its applicability to our present situation. The text of the Commission takes two examples from the Old Testament, regarding food prohibitions, to clarify this point. Finally, the persistence with which a moral theme appears in diverse texts points to its importance or abiding significance. The privileged concern for the poor, for example, responds to this criterion of persistence. This 'theme is to be found from one end of Scripture to the other'.[38]

The process of discernment cannot be limited to exegesis but must engage with the community of faith. *Community discernment*[39] is, therefore, an essential element of the dialogue between Scripture and moral reflection. The New Testament has given us a model of ecclesial discernment in Acts 15:1-35. The problem confronting the community of believers and recorded in Acts was a new one: whether Gentiles who had opted to become Christian were obliged to undergo circumcision. The narrative in Acts distinguishes three essential components of prudent discernment: a shared process, the search for a solution and a decision. The model of discernment acted out in this incident in the life of the early Church was essentially a spiritual discernment since it occurred in the context of debate and prayer (Acts 15:28).

The final element of discernment is that of *personal discernment*.⁴⁰ We are each ultimately called and enlightened by the Holy Spirit to discern conscientiously before making moral decisions. In this regard, Paul is presented to us as a model of personal discernment. In 1 Corinthians 8:1–11:1, he wrestled with an issue that was causing difficulties in the community: could Christians, without troubling their consciences, eat meat consecrated in sacrifice to idols and sold in the marketplace? As a result of his prayerful discernment, he concluded, in this particular context, love can compel us to renounce a right and to rectify our behaviour by taking into consideration the 'weak conscience' of others in order to avoid scandal. Paul's personal discernment is also evident in another difficult text (1 Cor 7:1-39), which wrestled with the implications of marriage between a believer and a non-believer, the significance of virginity and the significance of sexual abstinence for spiritual reasons amongst those who are married.

This last criterion of discernment emphasises the necessity of honouring the nature of biblical texts and avoiding a fundamentalist use of Scripture that, for example, isolates a biblical precept from its historical, cultural and literary context. It also highlights the important role of a living faith community in discerning the role of particular biblical texts in moral reflection. Finally, it acknowledges the indispensable role of personal prayerful discernment in the often difficult task of moral decision-making.

The reflections at the beginning of this chapter and the criteria proposed by the Pontifical Biblical Commission have attempted to tease out the role of Scripture in moral reflection and decision-making within the faith community. The criteria advanced by the Commission enable us to approach the Scriptures with greater confidence in our search for moral norms. They alert us to, among other things, the gradual unfolding of moral wisdom in the Scriptures and the importance of prayerful discernment by the individual believer and the community. Furthermore, the fundamental criteria proposed – the normative example of Christ and the biblical understanding of the person – give a stance on reality that has obvious implications for moral reflection.

Our first font of wisdom, Scripture, gives us a worldview or context out of which Christians engage in moral reflection. Scripture gives us an understanding of ourselves and of the world we live in that is unique and proposes Christ as the norm and model for humankind. We are called to allow the person and teaching of Christ and the message of the parables to shape our characters and actions.

2. Christian Tradition

For over two thousand years the Christian tradition has reflected on the nature and implications of becoming a 'new creation' in Christ. The fruits of this reflection are to be found in many places, including the liturgy and prayer life of the community, in Christian families and the 'sense of the faithful, and in the teaching of the Church. There are two important elements of this tradition that must be emphasised. In the first place, the tradition is dynamic and ongoing rather than static and complete. Because the Christian family is a *living* family of faith, it is continually bringing the Gospel into dialogue with changing cultures and situations. It must continue to read the 'signs of the times' in order to tease out the implications of the Gospel in ever-changing circumstances. In that sense, it is dynamic and open to new and deeper insights into the Gospel and its implications for humankind. The Church's stance on religious freedom in society or its appreciation of the value and role of women are good examples of how the Church's understanding of the Gospel and its implications for society deepened and matured over the centuries.[41]

Secondly, it is important to appreciate that the tradition of the Church – what it sees as important, life-giving and Gospel-focused – is witnessed to and lived out by the whole Church, including families, Christian organisations, prayer groups, Christian artists, theologians and those involved in ministry. They all witness and contribute to the ethos or fabric of the Christian life. They are all called and enabled to discern, with the help of the Holy Spirit, the demands of the Gospel in a changing world. Within this living tradition there is a special role for the teaching authority of the Church, the Magisterium, in proclaiming and teaching the truths and implications of the Christian faith.

The living tradition of the Church is a rich source of wisdom and insight into what constitutes right living. The rich corpus of Church teaching reminds us that generations before us have reflected on the central concerns of human identity – the nature of marriage, the demands of justice, the content of human rights – and that this source of wisdom is there for us to engage with and apply to our own contexts and circumstances. The Christian family is the bearer of a moral tradition that ensures that every new generation of the faith community does not have to reinvent the wheel! In the course of this book, we will draw heavily from the insights already formulated within the tradition on significant moral issues like euthanasia and reproductive technologies.

Several important questions, however, arise concerning the role of the Magisterium and the content of its teachings on moral and doctrinal issues. These include questions concerning the relationship between the individual person and the teaching authority of the Catholic faith community. In particular, questions arise as to the nature and role of individual conscience. How should individuals and their conscience relate to Church teaching? Questions also arise as to the different kinds of Church teaching in the area of morality and the various levels of authority and certitude associated with them. Finally, the relationship between Church teaching and the ethos of society, including the content of the civil law, needs to be explored and clarified. These important concerns and questions will be studied in chapters six and seven.

3. The Law of Reason: Natural Law

The third source of wisdom used to aid Christians in moral reflection is the natural law or law of reason.[42] The Catholic theological tradition has always maintained that God created humanity, but did not abandon it to a futile search for the meaning of life and the content of morality. Rather, the tradition argues, God both created humanity and endowed humanity with reason that enabled it to reflect on life and, through such reflection, discern the moral law. At the heart of the natural law tradition is the belief that, as rational beings, we can discern the difference between right and wrong by observing the world we inhabit and by reflecting on our experiences. Scholars note that St Paul (Rom 1:20; 2:14-16) recognised this fact when he claimed that pagans knew God's law because it was written on their hearts. Central to this tradition is a positive understanding of God and a positive understanding of the human person. We were endowed by God with reason in order to understand the world we live in and to discern what contributes to human flourishing. Thomas Aquinas provided a definition of the natural law that has endured in the tradition:

> The natural law is nothing other than the light of understanding placed in us by God; through it we know what we must do and what we must avoid. God has given this light or law at the creation.[43]

The natural law or the law of reason lies at the heart of the human rights tradition. That tradition claims that we can, through reflecting on the human person and our experiences, discern rights that are both intrinsic to the person and universal. The important thing to note here is that we discern these rights based on rational discernment and independent of any special divine revelation.

The strength of the natural law tradition is that it enables a universal discourse on what is ethical and leading to human happiness. People, independently of their religious convictions, can join together in the shared task of discerning what is good or right. This was always an important aspect and implication of the natural law tradition. This aspect is even more important today with societies being more religiously pluralistic. If everyone in society spoke only out of their own sacred texts – the Christian Bible or the Qur'an, for example – dialogue and shared initiatives would be very difficult. For this reason, Pope John Paul II and Pope Benedict XVI have spoken in recent times about the importance of the natural law tradition and the need for its renewal. In particular, the Magisterium and Catholic theologians see the natural law tradition as a valuable counterpoint to moral relativism and moral scepticism.[44] These related thought systems hold that all moral claims are of equal significance. Consequently, each person's understanding of the truth is valid, and the search for an objective, universally-binding morality is deemed unimportant or unattainable. Moral scepticism in particular denies the possibility of knowing the objective truth about life and its ultimate meaning. The best we can achieve, it argues, is some partial, provisional or subjective understanding of morality. They argue that moral knowledge, since it is mediated through experience, is always subjective and, therefore, incapable of being universalised.

In contrast to these movements, the natural law tradition boldly proclaims that there is an objective meaning or purpose to life and that this meaning can be grasped and understood through reasoned reflection.

Other critics of the natural law tradition claim that it is far too optimistic and doesn't take adequate account of the human condition. Many within the Reformed tradition hold this view; original sin damaged reason to such an extent that reason is not a reliable guide in the task of discerning God's ways. For this reason, they argued that Scripture (*Sola Scriptura*) is the only reliable source of moral wisdom. This understanding also found its way into parts of the Catholic moral tradition. The followers of Jansenism, for example, argued that Scripture and the Patristics were the only reliable guides for moral behaviour. Against this understanding, the Catholic tradition has always maintained that, despite original sin and its abiding effects, humans retain their rationality and can still discern the essentials of God's law. The tradition does acknowledge, however, that there are several obstacles or impediments that can make such discernment difficult.

'The precepts of the natural law are not perceived by everyone clearly and immediately.'[45] Sin, for example, can make us self-focused and unable to see clearly the demands of the moral law. Fear or ignorance, likewise, can diminish our ability to see and discern clearly. The dominant ethos or culture of society can also blind us to the demands of the moral law. Finally, poverty or the struggle to survive can compromise our ability to discern the 'good' in any particular situation. However, despite this acknowledgement of the difficulties inherent in discerning God's ways, the Catholic moral tradition retains its optimism in the ability of humanity, through reasoned reflection, to discern the difference between right and wrong.

A continuing challenge in the natural law tradition is that of teasing out how faith impacts on reason. This is a complex issue that has been studied by theologians and the Magisterium over many centuries.[46] It is sufficient for our present purposes to say that Christian faith informs, helps and enlightens reason.[47] Faith and revelation assist, rather than replace, reason by helping it to see clearly what reason unaided may, at times, only dimly see.

Finally, it would be disingenuous not to acknowledge that the natural law tradition has had, at times, a difficult history in the life of the Church. We can readily identify two factors that contributed to this difficult history. Over the course of history there have been, in the first place, conflicting understandings and applications of the natural law. These tensions and disagreements have been well documented and debated within the theological tradition.[48] It is argued that, in the area of sexual morality especially, the natural law was often understood as the law of nature rather than the law of reason. This lead to an approach to human sexuality that was seen by many to be inadequate. A second source of disagreement among theologians and others was in the unpacking of the notion of the natural law. The existence of a natural law was affirmed, but then many theologians and Church documents, immediately and with confidence, asserted that they knew exactly the content of the natural law. If only it was so simple! The reality is that the unpacking of the natural law, like the unpacking of the concept of human rights, is an ongoing task that demands patience, dialogue and modesty in one's claims. This is particularly true when it comes to discerning the 'small print' of the natural law. Today much scholarly work continues to be done both on the history of natural law and on its continued relevance for contemporary society.[49]

In this initial chapter, we have identified and examined the three sources of wisdom that the Catholic moral tradition utilises in the process of moral reflection. The Christian Scriptures provide the 'eyes' through which we understand ourselves and our place in the world and introduce us to the person and teachings of Christ. This source provides believers with the worldview or context out of which they deliberate on moral questions. The criteria provided by the Biblical Commission enable the moral teaching of the Scriptures to be responsibly and adequately engaged. The living faith community of the Church has reflected for over two thousand years on the meaning of life and has identified, in teachings, rituals and prayers, virtues and actions that conform to our nature and enable human flourishing. This source provides us with a rich inheritance that enables ongoing moral reflection. Finally, the natural law tradition recognises that as rational beings we can, by reflecting on experience, identify what contributes to human well-being. This tradition also enables people of good will everywhere to cooperate in the shared search for the truth about the human person and human flourishing.

In the following chapter, I will draw upon these sources as I examine a range of contemporary issues in the area of bioethics. These sources or fonts of wisdom will enable us to engage in a coherent process of moral reflection leading to credible moral conclusions.

DISCUSSION QUESTIONS
1. In the process of moral reflection, how useful are the Scriptures? What are the dangers to be avoided when using the Scriptures for moral reflection?

2. What are the benefits of the natural law tradition in religiously pluralistic societies?
3. If moral reflection is a function of reason, why are there so many conflicts worldwide on moral issues?
4. The Church is a dynamic community of faith with a living tradition about what is moral and important in life. Within the faith community, who should contribute to the ongoing task of discerning the demands of the Gospel?

FURTHER READING

Bretzke, James T., *A Morally Complex World*, Liturgical Press, 2004, chapters 2 and 3.

Gula, Richard, *Reason Informed by Faith*, Paulist Press, 1989, chapters 12, 13, 14, 15 and 16.

Hannon, Patrick, *Moral Decision Making*, Veritas, 2005, chapters 7, 8 and 9.

Harrington, Daniel and James Keenan, *Jesus and Virtue Ethics: Building Bridges Between New Testament Studies and Moral Theology*, Sheed & Ward, 2002.

MacNamara, Vincent, *The Call to be Human*, Veritas, 2010, chapters 5, 6, 7 and 8.

Pontifical Biblical Commission, *The Bible and Morality: Biblical Roots of Christian Conduct*, Libreria Editrice Vaticana, 2008.

NOTES

1. Pope John Paul II, *Evangelium vitae*, Veritas, 1995, paragraph 65.
2. Daniel Harrington and James Keenan, *Jesus and Virtue Ethics: Building Bridges Between New Testament Studies and Moral Theology*, Sheed & Ward, 2002; James T. Bretzke, *A Morally Complex World*, Liturgical Press, 2004, chapter 3; James Keating (ed.), *Moral Theology: New Directions and Fundamental Issues*, Paulist Press, 2004, chapters 2 and 5; Enda McDonagh and Vincent MacNamara (eds), *An Irish Reader in Moral Theology*, Columba Press, 2009, part 1.

3. Pontifical Biblical Commission, *The Bible and Morality: Biblical Roots of Christian Conduct*, Libreria Editrice Vaticana, 2008.
4. Pope Benedict XVI, *Caritas in veritate*, Veritas, 2009. See also *The Compendium of the Social Doctrine of the Church*, Veritas, 2004, chapter 10.
5. Ibid., paragraph 48. The Irish Catholic Bishops' Conference engaged with this text in their recent publication, *The Cry of the Earth: A Pastoral Reflection on Climate Change*, 2009.
6. Pontifical Biblical Commission, *The Bible and Morality*, paragraphs 95–99. The Commission identified the first fundamental criterion as 'conformity with the biblical concept of human nature'.
7. It is equally true that we are unlike God. Our 'non-likeness' to God is addressed in Pope John Paul II's *Mulieris dignitatem*, Veritas, 1988, paragraph 8.
8. For a critique of consumerism, see Pope John Paul II, *Centesimus annus*, paragraph 36; Pontifical Council for Justice and Peace, *Compendium of the Social Doctrine of the Church*, paragraph 360.
9. 'Solidarity highlights in a particular way the intrinsic social nature of the human person, the equality of all in dignity and rights and the common path of individuals and peoples towards an ever more committed unity.' *Compendium of the Social Doctrine of the Church*, paragraph 192.
10. The consequences of this change – from mutuality to domination – for humanity and, in particular, for women, is developed in Pope John Paul II's, *Mulieris dignitatem*, Veritas, 1988, chapter 4. See especially paragraph 10.
11. *The Bible and Morality*, paragraphs 100–103. The Commission identifies the second fundamental criterion as 'conformity with the example of Christ'.
12. Ibid., paragraphs 142–221.
13. Ibid., paragraph 145.
14. Ibid., paragraph 147.
15. Ibid., paragraph 148.
16. Ibid., paragraph 150.
17. Ibid., paragraph 152.
18. Ibid., paragraphs 154–155.
19. Ibid., paragraph 156.
20. Ibid., paragraphs 156–158.
21. Ibid., paragraphs 158–159.
22. Ibid., paragraph 159.
23. Ibid., paragraph 162.

24. Ibid., paragraphs 167–168.
25. Ibid., paragraphs 168–172.
26. Ibid., paragraph 173.
27. Ibid., paragraph 174.
28. Ibid., paragraph 178.
29. Ibid., paragraphs 180–183.
30. Ibid., paragraphs 183–185.
31. Ibid., paragraphs 185–186.
32. Ibid., paragraph 189.
33. Ibid., paragraph 191.
34. Ibid., paragraph 198.
35. Ibid., paragraph 208.
36. Ibid.
37. Ibid., paragraph 209.
38. Ibid., paragraph 212.
39. Ibid., paragraphs 213–215.
40. Ibid., paragraphs 216–218.
41. On the question of change and development in Church teaching, see John T. Noonan, *A Church That Can and Cannot Change*, University of Notre Dame Press, 2005; Charles E. Curran (ed.), *Change in Official Catholic Moral Teachings: Readings in Moral Theology No. 13*, Paulist Press, 2003.
42. *Catechism of the Catholic Church*, paragraphs 1954–1960.
43. St Thomas Aquinas, *Collationes in Decem, praeceptis 1*. See also Summa 1-11, Q. 91, Article 2, 'Natural law is nothing else than the rational creature's participation in the eternal law.'
44. Pope John Paul II, *Veritatis splendor*, Catholic Truth Society, 1993, paragraph 1.
45. *Catechism of the Catholic Church*, paragraph 1960.
46. Pope John Paul 11, *Fides et ratio*, Veritas, 1998.
47. The title of Richard Gula's book is revealing: *Reason Informed by Faith*. Faith does not supplant reason or trump it, but informs and enlightens it.
48. Richard Gula, *Reason Informed by Faith*, Paulist Press, 1989, chapters 15 and 16.
49. Jean Porter, *Natural and Divine Law: Reclaiming the Tradition for Christian Ethics*, William B. Eerdmans Publishing, 1999; Charles E. Curran and Richard McCormick SJ (eds), *Readings in Moral Theology No. 7*, Paulist Press, 1991.

Section Two

The Content of Catholic Moral Teaching

2   Assisted Human Reproduction

OVER THE PAST DECADES, THERE HAS BEEN AN INCREASE in the occurrence of childlessness in the world, particularly in the Western world. Several different reasons have been proposed to explain this phenomenon, including couples postponing starting a family until their mid-thirties; the use of the contraceptive pill over many years; and the presence of increasing amounts of additives in our diet. For many couples, this experience is the source of great heartbreak and disappointment. The scientific and medical community have responded to this reality by both investigating the causes of childlessness and striving to overcome it through direct intervention.

Louise Brown, in 1978, was the first person born through in vitro fertilisation (IVF) and since then there has been a phenomenal increase in the availability and variety of reproductive technologies. All countries in the European Union, including Ireland, now offer a range of reproductive technologies that enable couples who previously could not have children to have a family of their own. In some countries, legislation allows for the donation of genetic material and embryos and for the treatment of women who are post-menopause. These technologies raise important ethical, social and legal questions that previous generations never had to ponder: What is the nature of human parenthood? Is there a right to have a child? Should science enable women to procreate beyond the age of menopause? Does the donation of genetic material (sperm, ova or embryo) have an impact on our understanding of parenthood? What value or status should we give to human life at the earliest stage of its development? Is the fertilised ova deserving of more respect inside the womb than outside of it? What impact does surrogacy have on the well-being of a child? How do we evaluate human actions that are motivated by the best of intentions and yield positive consequences? These questions are important ones that have serious implications for individuals and societies. For this reason, many countries established select committees to investigate the ethics of reproductive technologies. The reports published by these groups often provided the framework and foundation for legislation in this area. One of the best known of these reports is the Warnock Report, which provided the framework for legislation in Britain.

Ireland, surprisingly, is one of the few countries that have failed to produce legislation to regulate the various aspects of reproductive technologies. These technologies are now only regulated in Ireland by the codes of conduct of the various medical professions involved. A Commission on Assisted Human Reproduction was established by the Irish Government in March 2000 to identify the central ethical, social and legal issues and to make recommendations on the content of civil legislation in this area. This Commission issued its report in April 2005.[1] The Commission made over forty recommendations governing the whole area of the regulation of assisted human reproduction.[2] At the time of writing, this report has not been acted upon and Ireland is still without legislation in this important area.

The Response of the Catholic Moral Tradition

The questions raised by the advances in reproductive technologies are important ones. They challenge us to reflect on issues that are at the core of our humanity. Because of the importance of these questions, the Catholic moral tradition, at both the universal and local level, has engaged with them in a serious and reflective way. At the level of the universal Church, these reflections were first articulated in *Donum vitae*,[3] published nine years after the birth of Louise Browne. Later publications of the universal Magisterium built on the moral analysis of this document.[4] Local Churches, including the Irish Church, have developed their own responses in light of this universal teaching.[5]

The basic building block of many of the new technologies is in vitro fertilisation (IVF). This process involves the surgical removal of ova (by laparoscopy) and their mixing with sperm. Once fertilisation has occurred, the developing embryo is placed in the uterine cavity to continue its journey towards maturity. In most fertility programmes many ova are fertilised, three are usually implanted and the surplus embryos are used in a variety of ways. Since the success rate of IVF is still modest, many couples have to repeat the procedure before the successful birth of a child. To facilitate this possibility, and to avoid a repeat laparoscopy, surplus embryos are frozen in a significant number of cases. These can be retrieved if, and when, the need arises.

A second possible use of these surplus embryos involves their donation to other couples. This eventuality could arise if, for a host of reasons, a woman/couple could not create an embryo but could successfully carry an embryo to birth.

Finally, many jurisdictions allow for the donation of surplus embryos to the scientific community for research purposes. Such research, it is argued, could benefit the human family by yielding information about infertility and the life of the early embryo.[6] The use of such embryos to advance stem cell research will be examined in the next chapter.

In their response to the developments in reproductive technologies over the past thirty years, ethicists have made some general points that are worth noting. Firstly, ethicists and the science of ethics would reject what is called 'the scientific imperative'. This is formulated in many different ways but its essence is transparent in the following phrase: 'If we *can* do it, then we *must* do it'. The discipline of ethics, in contrast, raises the 'ought we' question; just because, as a consequence of newfound knowledge and expertise, we can do something new and exciting, does not answer the question of whether we should do it.[7]

Secondly, ethicists alert us to the reality that there can be a difference between scientific progress and human progress. Advances in the area of science and technology need not necessarily contribute to the progress of the human family. The development of atomic weaponry and 'Star Wars' technology clearly illustrate this distinction. Though they are the fruits of undoubted human genius and creativity, they have not contributed to the flourishing of the human family.

Discussions amongst ethicists on the merits of reproductive technologies have also highlighted the fact that individuals can approach the task of making moral decisions from very different perspectives. The robust debates in the area of bioethics over the past few decades have, with great clarity, revealed that our approach to the task of moral decision-making has a decisive impact on our moral conclusions.

Before proceeding further, therefore, I will first engage with the question of moral decision-making. In particular, I will look at the role of object, intention and circumstance in determining the morality of human actions.

The Evaluation of Human Actions

Individuals and communities everywhere acknowledge that the birth of a child is a positive and graced event. The child born through IVF is, like all children, a child of God and a bearer of an innate dignity. As such s/he is to be respected and loved unconditionally. However, the Catholic tradition argues that there is an obligation on us to examine the *means* used to achieve the undeniable good that is the birth of a child.

The Christian tradition has reflected over many centuries, and in various cultural contexts, on the roots of morality. One of the fruits of this sustained reflection and study is the acceptance of the principle that 'the end does not justify the means'. Consequently, there is a need in this context, as in all others, to examine the process of IVF in a systematic and objective way.

The Catholic tradition's rejection of the 'end justifies the means' approach to morality begs the question, how then does one evaluate human actions? In response to this central question, the Catholic moral tradition has embraced what is called the three-font principle.[8] In this understanding there are three dimensions of a human act that need to be examined in order to get an adequate picture of the act. These are the act in itself (*finis operis*), the intention of the person doing the act (*finis operantis*) and the circumstances, including consequences, of the act. Consideration of all three is necessary in order to get an accurate picture of what is going on in any human drama.

A few simple examples should help clarify this approach. Hitting your neighbour with your fist (act in itself) is an action that requires further detail before we have a full picture of the scene and before we can arrive at a moral judgement. Was the action motivated by hatred and with the intention of causing harm? Or was it motivated by the legitimate need to defend oneself from an unwarranted assault while doing the least physical harm necessary to achieve that goal? These very different scenarios, defined by the intention of the agent and the circumstances, lead us to very different moral conclusions. Likewise, for most people, the taking of human life is evaluated in light of intention and circumstances. Thus, killing another person in war or in self-defence, under certain circumstances, is deemed morally acceptable to most people.

The Catholic moral tradition maintains that other approaches to the moral evaluation of human actions are inadequate because they neglect to take into account vital aspects of the unfolding drama. These include ethical systems that focus exclusively either on the *intention* of the actor or the *consequences* of the action. At the heart of many current debates in society on the morality of specific actions is this underlying disagreement about how to approach the task of moral evaluation. The conclusions of the Catholic moral tradition are often at odds with the conclusions of others precisely because of this fundamental disagreement about method.

For the sake of completion it is important to mention that there are, in the Catholic moral tradition, a collection of human actions that can be evaluated outside of this three-font (object, intention, circumstance) approach. These have traditionally been called *intrinsically evil acts* and have been defined as actions that are in themselves (*per se*) and independently of circumstances and intention always wrong.[9] These actions are always and everywhere wrong because by their very nature they are contrary to the dignity of the person and an affront to God. Traditionally, lying and adultery were listed as such acts. The *Catechism of the Catholic Church* includes blasphemy, perjury and murder in this category.[10] This way of categorising human actions is not, however, unproblematic and has been the subject of much theological discussion. There is no disputing the fact that there are many actions that are always immoral. Disagreement amongst theologians centres on the usefulness and coherence of the intrinsically evil category. Unfortunately, the range of actions listed under this category in the *Catechism of the Catholic Church* and in *Veritatis splendor* did nothing to contribute to clarity on the issue, since some of them appear as tautologies.[11] This discussion amongst theologians, though important and interesting, need not detain us further. What is important for our purposes is that the Catholic moral tradition insists that three aspects of a human action must be taken into account before that action can be morally evaluated. Though those providing and availing of artificial reproductive technologies are motivated by generosity and love, we still need to look at the procedure itself before we can arrive at a moral evaluation. In particular, we need to reflect on, in the first place, the status and fate of the fertilised ovum, because it is the building block on which reproductive technologies are built and, secondly, on the significance of generating life without bodily intercourse. These two aspects of reproductive technologies were central to the analysis and conclusions of *Donum vitae* and later documents.

THE STATUS OF THE FERTILISED OVUM
The process of IVF raises the question about the significance of human life at its beginning. In a dramatic way we can now observe the earliest stages of life in the palm of our hand. What value or significance should we give to life at this stage? This is, in one sense, a new question. Previous generations

did reflect on the value of life in the womb but never encountered the beginning of life in such a dramatic way.

Debates across the globe about the value or significance of human life at the earliest stages have generated much passion but, unfortunately, little agreement. Philosophers, theologians, politicians and legal systems hold a range of positions on this vital question. In the Irish context, for example, the Supreme Court in December 2009 ruled that the pre-implanted (frozen) embryo does not have the protection of the Constitution under Article 40.3.3.[12] That article, amended in 1983, requires 'the State to respect and vindicate the right to life of the unborn with due regard to the equal right to life of the mother'. The case arose when a couple, whose marriage had ended, disagreed about the fate of frozen embryos that they had created. These embryos were frozen during an earlier successful IVF treatment cycle. The mother in the case wanted the embryos implanted in her and brought to full term. The father, on the basis that they were no longer a couple, did not agree with that proposal. In deciding on what was a complex case on many fronts, the Courts had to make a determination as to the status of frozen, pre-implanted embryos.

The Supreme Court, upholding a High Court decision in 2006, ruled that pre-implanted embryos are not 'unborn' within the meaning of Article 40. The Constitution, under Article 40.3.3, it ruled, grants protection only to embryos within the womb.[13] On the basis of this judgement, embryos are treated differently by the civil law in Ireland depending on whether they are within or outside the womb. This has important implications for the future treatment of pre-implanted embryos in Irish fertility programmes.

The Catholic tradition has, over the last century, articulated an approach to the human embryo that is both consistent and credible. It argues that human life should be protected and revered from the beginning of its existence. It accepts that at fertilisation something new comes into existence that is biologically human, different from the ovum and sperm from which it originated, and containing all the genetic material necessary to develop into a person or persons. After fertilisation nothing new is added to the genetic package of this new living entity. The tradition accepts the evidence of the biological sciences that early human life goes through a whole range of developments from zygote to embryo to foetus. However, it argues that life should be protected, valued and treasured equally during all these stages and that a 'gradation in moral value'[14] is unacceptable. It is worth noting at this stage that the Irish Council for Bioethics in their publication on stem cell research, which will be examined in the next chapter, adopted this 'gradualist position' to the status of the embryo.[15] For its part, the Warnock Report proposed the 'primitive streak' as the stage of development that is most significant in terms of moral status. At this stage the cells of the early embryo became differentiated and assume a definite shape around a central axis.

Many contributors to the debate on the significance of human life at the very beginning of its development utilise the language of person. Some argue that because only a person can be the bearer of human rights, including the right to life and the right to be free from assault, the central question to be addressed is whether, or when, the embryo becomes a person. If the embryo is not a person, so the argument runs, then the question of its treatment or destruction is not problematic from a moral perspective. How has the Catholic moral tradition responded to this approach? Does it believe that the newly fertilised ovum is a person and, therefore, a bearer of rights? *Donum vitae* acknowledges that the question of personhood is a difficult and complex one. Questions about the nature and scope of personhood spring easily to mind: What is necessary to become a person? Is a newborn baby a person? Can personhood be lost through a debilitating illness or serious injury? *Donum vitae* does not take a position on the various philosophical approaches to the nature and content of human personhood. Rather, it argues that being a member of the human family is synonymous with personhood. It asks rhetorically, 'How could a human individual not be a human person?'[16] Given that the fertilised ova is biologically human, and has its own unique genetic package to direct its future development, it argues that it should be treated 'as a person' from the first moment of its existence. Consequently, the rights of the embryo, among which, 'in the first place, is the inviolable right of every innocent human being to life'[17] must be recognised. The latest text from the Congregation for the Doctrine of the Faith, *Dignitas personae*, adopts a similar approach, arguing that the 'human embryo has from the very beginning the dignity proper to a person'.[18]

With regard to reproductive programmes that utilise IVF, this understanding has significant consequences. If our starting point is that human life is deserving of respect from the first moment of its existence, then several features of many reproductive programmes appear unethical. The discarding of 'surplus embryos', the manipulation of embryos or their donation for research purposes are all inconsistent with respect for human life.[19] It can, indeed, be argued that these practices contribute to an erosion of respect for human life at all its stages. They contribute to a culture that places little value on human life at the earliest stages of its development. From a Catholic Christian perspective, which believes that all life should be treasured and valued because it is a gift from God, this culture is seriously flawed.

Using the sources of moral wisdom, outlined in chapter one, we see that the Church's approach to and moral conclusions about the treatment of the embryo are rooted in Scripture (the general call to respect the gift of life), reason (what science tells us about the fertilised ovum) and tradition (the consistent stance of the Church and the faith community on respect for human life).

The Nature of Human Procreation

The second pillar on which the Catholic tradition constructs its response to IVF and other reproductive technologies is that of its understanding of human sexuality and the nature of human procreation. *Donum vitae* begins its reflection on the process of IVF and, in particular, on the fact that fertilisation, leading to procreation, is achieved without bodily intercourse with a question: 'What connection is required from the moral point of view between procreation and the conjugal act?'[20]

It constructs its response to this question using three distinct, but somewhat overlapping, arguments. The first argument is based on the nature of human sexuality as understood in the Catholic moral tradition. It is self-evident that through our sexuality and sexual expression we express both love and affection and can generate new life. Our sexuality has both love-expressing and life-creating dimensions. Church teaching, however, goes further than this and 'affirms the "inseparable connection, willed by God and unable to be broken by man on his own initiative, between the two meanings of the conjugal act: the unitive meaning and the procreative meaning".'[21]

This understanding of the nature of human sexuality is, of course, central to the teaching of *Humanae vitae*. In that document it was argued that we should not engage in physical lovemaking other than in an environment that is not closed to new life. We should not intentionally and directly exclude the procreative dimension if that dimension is naturally present.

Donum vitae, using the same framework of understanding, argues from the other side of the coin. While *Humanae vitae* argues that we should not deliberately remove the procreative dimension of the conjugal act, *Donum vitae* argues that we should not procreate outside of physical lovemaking.

The implications of this understanding of human sexuality for family planning are, of course, well known. The insistence on the inseparability of the two dimensions of sexuality – the procreative and the unitive – has been criticised by many within, and outside, the Catholic tradition. Critics question, in particular, the inseparability argument. Why, it is asked, is it not permissible to use our skills and creativity to directly exclude the procreative dimension for serious personal or family reasons? Should not our potential to procreate be at the service of our relationships or families in their totality? The debate about the coherence and credibility of the moral conclusions of *Humanae vitae* on the use of artificial contraceptives has been well aired and documented over the past forty years. It is beyond the scope of this book to enter into the important theological debate generated by that document concerning, amongst other things, the natural law, moral method and ecclesiology. From the perspective of this book's treatment of bioethical issues, it is sufficient to note that the first argument used in *Donum vitae* works out of the framework of understanding of human sexuality found in *Humanae vitae*. The implication of the inseparability argument for in vitro fertilisation is crystal clear. Science may *assist* the conjugal act to achieve a pregnancy, but may not *replace* the conjugal act.[22]

The second argument presented in response to the question about the relationship between procreation and the conjugal act may appear to some people to be more robust and reasonable. This argument reflects on the significance of the human body. It argues that we are embodied creatures who express affection, love and marital commitment through our bodies. Our bodies and bodily gestures are an essential part of who we are.

> Spouses mutually express their personal love in the 'language of the body', which clearly involves both 'spousal meanings' and 'parental ones'. ... It is in their bodies and through their bodies that the spouses consummate their marriage and are able to become father and mother.[23]

By procreating outside of the context of bodily intercourse we are disrespecting, or, at least, not paying adequate attention to, our nature as bodily persons.

The third argument presented revolves around the dignity of the child created through IVF. It argues, firstly, that the child must be respected as an equal in dignity to the parents who gave him/her life. Secondly, it argues that the process of assisted human reproduction has implications for how we see or prize the child conceived. Every child should be the fruit of a loving conjugal act where 'the spouses cooperate as servants and not as masters in the work of the Creator who is love'.[24]

The important point being made here is that parents are called to cooperate with God in the act of procreation rather than dominate that process. The document goes on to argue:

> In reality, the origin of a human person is the result of an act of giving. The one conceived must be the fruit of his parents' love. He cannot be desired or conceived as the

product of an intervention of medical or biological techniques; that would be equivalent to reducing him to an object of scientific technology.[25]

Implicit in this argument is the claim that through controlling the process of procreation the child is not seen as a gift, but more as the end product of a process of control. The difference between the language of procreation and that of reproduction may throw some light on this claim. The former expression implies that humankind cooperate with God in the act of creating new life while the latter, in using the language of industry, emphasises human domination and control of the process. However, it is unclear from the text, and from human experience, how a child conceived through IVF and clearly wanted by his/her parents would be viewed as 'an object of scientific technology'. The argument appears, at best, strained and, at worst, incredible and, not surprisingly, does not appear in later documents.

The question of how we view the child conceived through IVF is touched on again later in the document, but in a more credible way. The context is a brief discussion on whether there is a right to have a child.

> Nevertheless, marriage does not confer upon the spouses the right to have a child, but only the right to perform those natural acts which are per se ordered to procreation. A true and proper right to a child would be contrary to the child's dignity and nature. The child is not an object to which one has a right.[26]

The important point being made here is that the language of rights is inappropriate in this area because it could contribute to a culture that views children as possessions or objects.

Because children are equal in dignity to their parents and all other persons, they cannot be instrumentalised in this way.

The second pillar on which the Church's response to artificial reproductive technologies is constructed is based on the Church's understanding of human sexuality and the nature of human parenthood, and leads it to reject procedures that *replace* the conjugal act, such as IVF, gamete intra-fallopian transfer (GIFT) and intra-cytoplasmic sperm injection (ICSI).[27] Procedures that, on the other hand, act as an aid to the conjugal act and its fertility – for example, surgery, drug treatment or NaPro technology – are permitted. The approach and conclusions of Church teaching in this regard are rooted loosely in Scripture (the significance of marriage as the locus for family), reason (the nature of human sexuality) and tradition (the consistent teaching of the Church).

Reproductive technologies have raised considerable questions for societies across the globe. These include questions concerning the status of human life at the earliest stage of development, the nature of human parenthood, the significance of our embodiment and the right to have a child. Societies worldwide have responded to these questions in a myriad of ways. This is reflected in the rich variety of legislative frameworks within which reproductive technologies are carried out.

During the (ongoing) debate on the ethics of reproductive technologies, the Catholic moral tradition has articulated a clear and consistent stance. It firmly argues that life should be treasured and protected from the moment of fertilisation, rather than at some later stage like implantation or at the appearance of the primitive streak. This position was clearly articulated in *Donum vitae* and appears even more prominently in later teaching documents.[28] It concludes, therefore, that discarding, freezing or experimenting with 'surplus' embryos is morally unacceptable. Such activities, it contends, contribute to an erosion of respect for pre-implanted life and contribute to a culture that sees human life at that early stage as of little value.

It strongly argues, also, that the nature of human parenthood is fundamentally contradicted by third party involvement in the form of surrogate mothers or donors of genetic material. In its understanding of the Christian vision and the natural law tradition, parenthood is the prerogative of married couples. As for the process itself, whereby fertilisation is achieved without sexual intercourse, it argues that it does not adequately respect the nature of human sexuality or our reality as bodily persons. Finally, the tradition suggests that reproductive technologies can alter the ways we experience and value children – a move from accepting children as a gift from God to a mindframe that views children as a right.

DISCUSSION QUESTIONS
1. 'The human being is to be respected and treated as a person from the first moment of conception.' Is this moral claim countercultural or mistaken?
2. 'It is in their bodies and through their bodies that the spouses consummate their marriage and are able to become father and mother.' Why should we procreate through bodily intercourse only?
3. Is there a right to have a child?

FURTHER READING
Ashley, Benedict, and Kevin O'Rourke (eds), *Ethics of Healthcare* (Third Edition), Georgetown University Press, 2002, chapter 9.
Congregation for the Doctrine of the Faith, *Donum vitae*, Veritas, 1987.
———, *Dignitas personae*, Veritas, 2009.
Irish Catholic Bishops' Conference, *Assisted Human Reproduction: Facts and Ethical Issues*, Veritas, 2000.

———, *Towards a Creative Response to Infertility*, Veritas, 2006.
Sutton, Agneta, *Christian Bioethics: A Guide for the Perplexed*, Continuum, 2008, chapter 2.
Watt, Helen, *Life and Death in Healthcare Ethics: A Short Introduction*, Routledge, 2000, chapter 5.

NOTES

1. *Report of the Commission on Assisted Human Reproduction*, April, 2005. The text is available on the Department of Health and Children website: www.dohc.ie.
2. For a response to these recommendations, see Pádraig Corkery, 'Reproductive Technologies – The Irish Contribution to an International Debate', *The Furrow*, 56 (2005), pp. 353–357; Irish Catholic Bishops' Conference, *Towards a Creative Response to Infertility*, Veritas, 2006.
3. Congregation for the Doctrine of the Faith, *Donum vitae*, Libreria Editrice Vaticana, 1987.
4. Pope John Paul II, *Evangelium vitae*, Veritas, 1995, paragraph 63; Congregation for the Doctrine of the Faith, *Dignitas personae: On Certain Bioethical Issues*, Veritas, 2009; Pope Benedict XVI, *Caritas in veritate*, Veritas, 2009, paragraph 51.
5. Bishop's Committee on Bioethics, *Assisted Human Reproduction: Facts and Ethical Issues*, Veritas, 2000; Irish Catholic Bishops' Conference, *Towards a Creative Response to Infertility*, Veritas, 2006.
6. See, for example, the *Report of the Commission on Assisted Human Reproduction*, Recommendation No. 10: 'Appropriate guidelines should be put in place by the regulatory body to govern the options available for excess frozen embryos. These should include voluntary donation of excess healthy embryos to other recipients, voluntary donation for research or allowing them to perish.'
7. 'But what is technically possible is not for that very reason morally admissible.' Congregation for the Doctrine of the Faith, *Donum vitae*, Introduction, paragraph 4.
8. Richard Gula, *Reason Informed by Faith*, Paulist Press, 1989, chapter 18.
9. Pope John Paul II, *Veritatis splendor*, Veritas, 1993, paragraph 80.
10. *Catechism of the Catholic Church*, Veritas, 1994, paragraph 1756.

11. Murder, for example, is an unjustified killing. This judgement is made *after* the intention and circumstances have been taken into account. These considerations help us to distinguish murder from killing another in self-defence or accidental killing.
12. Roche v Roche. The full text of the Supreme Court judgment is available at www.courts.ie.
13. This position was proposed in the *Report of the Commission on Assisted Human Reproduction*, No. 16: 'The embryos formed by IVF should not attract legal protection until placed in the human body, at which stage it should attract the same level of protection as the embryo formed in vivo'.
14. Congregation for the Doctrine of the Faith, *Dignitas personae*, Veritas, 2009, paragraph 5.
15. The Irish Council for Bioethics, *Ethical, Scientific and Legal Issues Concerning Stem Cell Research: Opinion*, 2008, paragraph 41.
16. *Donum vitae*, chapter 1, question 1.
17. Ibid.
18. *Dignitas personae*, paragraph 5.
19. *Donum vitae*, chapter 1; *Dignitas personae*, paragraphs 14–16, 18–23.
20. *Donum vitae*, chapter 2, question 4.
21. *Donum vitae*, chapter 2, question 4, quoting *Humanae vitae*, paragraph 12.
22. *Dignitas personae*, paragraph 12.
23. *Donum vitae*, chapter 2, question 4.
24. Ibid.
25. Ibid.
26. Ibid., question 8.
27. Congregation for the Doctrine of the Faith, *Dignitas personae*, paragraph 12, 17; Irish Catholic Bishops' Conference, *Assisted Human Reproducton: Facts and Ethical Issues*, chapter 3.
28. For a view of the different emphases and approaches to reproductive technologies in the Irish context see Pádraig Corkery, 'Bio-ethics and Contemporary Irish Moral Discourse' in *Contemporary Irish Moral Discourse*, Amelia Fleming (ed.), Columba Press, 2007, pp. 26–39.

3 Embryonic Stem Cell Research

IN RECENT YEARS, FEW DEVELOPMENTS HAVE GENERATED as much excitement and discussion as stem cells and, particularly, stem cells derived from embryos. These, it is claimed by the scientific community, have the potential to make a very significant contribution to the health and well-being of the human family, both immediately and in the future. Stem cells are beneficial because, in non-scientific terms, they can be manipulated into becoming cells or, indeed, organs that are needed by individuals afflicted by a range of serious health issues. They are seen as a panacea for many of the most debilitating and distressing conditions that can afflict humanity.

Currently, embryos that are used for their stem cells come from two different sources. Fertility clinics worldwide produce many 'surplus' embryos that are no longer required by their genetic parents. These surplus embryos are often donated, rather than simply discarded, so that stem cells may be extracted from them. The second source is found in countries that allow for the creation of embryos for the *specific purpose* of scientific research. These embryos can be created through the usual process of IVF using donated genetic material. Alternatively, they can be created through cloning. The process of cloning is technically known as somatic cell nuclear transfer (SCNT). The process involves de-nucleating a female egg (ovum) and inserting into it the nucleus taken from a somatic (non-reproductive) cell of the person you want to clone. When an electric shock is applied the nucleus begins to develop into an embryo. The novelty factor here is that the embryo created has the genetic makeup of the owner of the somatic cell. For the first time in the history of humankind it is possible to create a human person who is not the fruit of two genetic inheritances (i.e. male and female), but only that of the somatic cell donor.[1] Given the reality of a steady stream of surplus embryos from fertility clinics, it is reasonable to ask why anyone would want to clone an embryo. In contemporary medicine, one of the problems associated with any kind of transplant is the fear of rejection. Scientists hope that, in some future time, they will be able to produce human blood, tissue and even organs by the use of stem cells. With the use of a cloned embryo the tissue and organs created would match the genetic makeup of the donor. This would, it is hoped, greatly reduce the difficulties associated with rejection. In theory, then, an individual could, through the use of an embryo clone of themselves, create blood, tissue and organs that would match their genetic profile and, therefore, reduce the possibility of rejection or other complications.

There are two different types of cloning: 'therapeutic' cloning and 'reproductive' cloning. 'Therapeutic' cloning occurs when an embryo is cloned in order to secure its stem cells. The extraction of the stem cells will, as always, lead to the destruction of the embryo. Cloning, in this case, is judged to be therapeutic because the future development of stem cell medicine will bring relief and possible cures to countless people. It is not, obviously, therapeutic for the embryo that has been created and destroyed. For this reason, the word 'therapeutic' seems inappropriate and, indeed, misleading.

'Reproductive' cloning, on the other hand, refers to the cloning of embryos in order to bring them to full term and birth. Nations across the world have specifically prohibited this development, though rogue scientists have claimed in the media to have accomplished this feat.

Finally, embryos can be created from human DNA and the egg of an animal. Scientists developed this technique because of the shortage of donated human female eggs. As a consequence of this shortage, they argued, research was hampered in this important area.

The genuine excitement that surrounds this area of scientific endeavour is accompanied by significant levels of controversy and moral disagreement among professional ethicists and within society at large. Given that embryonic stem cells have the potential to benefit humanity, now and in the future, and that the embryos are either donated or created under license, where, you may ask, is the ethical issue? Many people, indeed, argue that the donation of embryos or genetic material is a radical form of altruism, rather than an ethically controversial act, that has the potential to bring significant benefit to the human family. However, the use of embryonic stem cells continues to be controversial because the extraction of the stem cells causes the destruction of the embryo. This is an area of conflict because many people hold that the embryo has a significant status and that its direct destruction is morally unacceptable.[2] The approach and conclusion of the Catholic moral tradition to the issue of embryo destruction is clear-cut and has been outlined in the previous chapter. A second source of disagreement centres on the role given to (good) intentions and (good) consequences in moral decision-making. In the previous chapter, we saw that the Catholic moral tradition rejects as inadequate systems of moral analysis that focus exclusively on intention or consequences. It proposes instead the three-font principle as a coherent and credible framework for moral analysis.

It may be instructive to look at the ethical concerns raised by embryonic stem cell research by examining two Irish publications that made recommendations on legislation in this area. The Commission on Assisted Human Reproduction, which we were introduced to in the last chapter, made several recommendations pertinent to embryonic stem cell research, including:

> *No. 16* The embryos formed by IVF should not attract legal protection until placed in the human body, at which stage it should attract the same level of protection as the embryo formed in vivo. ...[3]

> *No. 34* Embryo research, including embryonic stem cell research, for specific purposes only and under stringently controlled conditions, should be permitted on surplus embryos that are donated specifically for research. This should be permitted up to fourteen days after fertilisation. ...[4]

> *No. 36* Regenerative (therapeutic cloning) medicine should be permitted under regulation.[5]

More recently, the Irish Council for Bioethics examined, in a systematic and thorough way, the many issues involved in embryonic stem cell research and made recommendations as to the shape of legislation and policies in this area.[6]

At the outset of its publication, the Bioethics Council noted the lack of legislation in Ireland in this area, despite the earlier Report of the Commission on Human Reproduction, and the resulting uncertainty about the legal status of the pre-implanted embryo.

From the many competing understandings on the moral status of the embryo, the Council adopted what it termed a 'gradualist position, granting significant moral value rather than full moral status to human embryos. The moral value they are seen to possess is based on recognition of their potential to develop into persons, as well as the value they derive from representing human life in its earliest stages'.[7] This understanding of the status of the embryo informs their moral assessment of, and recommendations for, embryonic stem cell research.

Their stance on the use of embryos from the first source, i.e. supernumerary IVF embryos, flows logically and consistently from this view of the moral status of the pre-implanted embryo. The Council, in its recommendations, supports the carefully regulated use of *supernumerary* IVF embryos – which are otherwise destined to be destroyed – for the purposes of embryonic stem cell research aimed at alleviating human suffering. The Council argued that, in the absence of definitive evidence that adult stem cells offer an equal or better prospect for developing therapies, embryonic stem cell research is 'a proportionate response to the needs of medical research'.[8] Furthermore, it insisted that the decision to donate supernumerary embryos for research 'should be voluntary, free from any form of coercion and made under the strict conditions of informed consent'.[9]

Also central to the Council's recommendations is an understanding that the value of human embryos that are surplus to IVF treatments needs to be balanced against 'the moral value of human welfare'.[10] From their perspective, it is a question of competing claims, respect for the embryo and concern for the alleviation of human suffering. In their judgement, the latter claim has more weight than the former.

On the important question of moral complicity and moral consistency – a subject of discussion following University College Cork's (UCC) decision to import embryonic stem cells for research purposes – the Council states that 'it has no objection to the use of therapies or the importation of stem cells derived from embryos'.[11] This conclusion is consistent with its own stance on the use of supernumerary embryos for stem cell research. Because the Council views such a use of embryos to be ethical, it has no objection to the importation of stem cells from this source or to benefiting from treatments derived from this source. However, instructively, it does acknowledge that 'benefiting from the use of embryonic stem cell lines or therapies derived from research one does not support raises serious considerations about moral consistency'.[12]

The notion of moral consistency raised by the Council is at the heart of the Catholic moral tradition's approach to cooperation and complicity in the wrongdoing of others. This principle, and recent uses of it, will be examined later in the chapter.

As indicated earlier, the second source of embryos for embryonic stem cell research is through the *creation* of embryos *specifically* for research purposes. The Council first examined the two methods most frequently used to create embryos: IVF and cloning (somatic cell nuclear transfer). The Council argued, in the first place, that a distinction should not be made between the moral status of an embryo created through the process of IVF and a cloned embryo. Therefore, it argued, the creation of embryos through IVF or somatic cell nuclear transfer for research purposes raise similar ethical issues. The Council concluded, however, that the creation of embryos specifically for research is not 'currently justified or represents a proportionate response while supernumerary IVF embryos exist'.[13]

It went on to argue, however, that should IVF processes become more efficient and, therefore, no longer a source of surplus embryos, or if the therapeutic potential of cloning (SCNT) is borne out by research, their conclusions 'may have to be re-evaluated'.[14]

Central to the approach and conclusions of the Council on the disputed issue of *creating* embryos for embryonic stem cell research was its desire to adopt the least morally offensive approach and to avoid the instrumentalisation of the embryo. It recognised that the creation of embryos specifically for research, which is dependent on the destruction of the embryo, is a very contentious issue worldwide. However, as already indicated, they were willing to revise their negative conclusion on the creation of embryos if supernumerary embryos were no longer available or if the use of cloned embryos were judged to bring significant therapeutic benefits. The significant moral weight they gave to the well-being of the human family trumped their concerns regarding the instrumentalisation of the embryo or the giving of moral offence. The *good consequences* of embryonic stem cell research and use for the human family featured decisively, then, in their moral analysis and conclusions. Consequently, they argued that if the creation of embryos was deemed necessary to achieve the good end of the well-being of the human family, they 'would have *no principled* objection to the creation of human-animal hybrid cell lines'.[15] Concerns surrounding the exploitation and coercion of women in the acquisition of human eggs also played an important role in their reflections on this issue.

Scientific literature has, over the past decade, also highlighted other sources of stem cells, including the umbilical cord, which is seen as a valuable and accessible source. Against this background the Council reflected on the merits of umbilical cord blood banking.[16] In their publication they argue that further scientific evidence and economic analyses are needed before a decision could be made regarding the benefits of such a scheme. Their recommendation, however, is that if such a system is constructed, it should follow a public, rather than a private, model of delivery.

On the important issue of patenting embryonic stem cells, the Council recorded its opposition based on the moral value it accorded the embryo and its unease with the instrumentalisation of human life.[17]

The Response of the Catholic Moral Tradition

The response of the Catholic tradition to the creation and use of embryonic stem cells is clear, consistent and grounded in a particular understanding of the significance of human life and the process of moral decision-making. On the basis of this framework of understanding, the approach and recommendations of the two Irish bodies outlined here are seriously flawed. The roots of their shortcomings lay in their stance on the status of the embryo and the role they assign to (good) intentions and (good) consequences in moral decision-making. Across the globe, similarly, those who support embryonic stem cell research either undervalue the embryo and/or give undue significance to good intentions and/or good consequences in their moral reasoning.

The response of the Catholic tradition to these Irish reports and to embryonic stem cell research in general follows the lines outlined in the previous chapter. For that reason they will be dealt with in summary form only. The acceptance of a gradualist approach to the status of the embryo, by the Council and others, impacts decisively on moral conclusions concerning a wide variety of issues. It allows for the destruction of the embryo on the basis of goals or goods that are deemed to be more significant. The starting point for the deliberation of the Catholic tradition, as outlined in *Donum vitae*, *Evangelium vitae* and *Dignitas personae*, is that the embryo – implanted or pre-implanted – is to be treated as a person from the beginning of its existence. As such, it is the bearer of rights, including the right to be free from destructive interventions. The direct and intentional destruction of the embryo is, consequently, seen as a grave offence against the gift of life.

The principle of the non-instrumentalisation of human life, utilised by the Council for Bioethics in some of its recommendations, is, in the Catholic tradition, applied to the embryo from the very beginning. The embryo should not, therefore, be used as an instrument to bring benefit to others. It cannot be treated as a 'means' to achieve an 'end', even when that 'end' is defined in terms of the present or future health of individuals or society.

Secondly, as outlined in the previous chapter, the tradition rejects as inadequate an approach to decision-making that focuses exclusively or decisively on the good consequences of a proposed action or the good intention of the doer of the act. In this particular case, many supporters of embryonic stem cell research argue primarily on these grounds: the many benefits that will accrue to the human family and the good intentions of all those involved. The tradition deems this to be inadequate because it fails to deal seriously with the object of the act.

In addition to these two central issues, the creation and destruction of *cloned* embryos and *hybrid* embryos raise additional moral and ethical issues that have profound implications for society and the common good.[18] In particular, the cloning of embryos raises serious questions about individuality, uniqueness and the limits of human stewardship of the gift of creation.

Moral Consistency and the Principle of Cooperation and Scandal

The decision of the authorities in University College Cork in 2009 to allow the importation of embryonic stem cells from abroad generated some discussion about moral consistency. In particular, opponents of the decision argued that to benefit from or participate in embryonic stem cell research involves cooperation with the wrongdoing of others. Such cooperation, they argued, amounts to complicity in the moral wrongdoing of others and is a morally inconsistent stance for those who have moral objections to the destruction of the embryo.

The questions raised by the decision of UCC to import stem cells derived from embryos are important and deserving of further reflection. If one's personal stance is that the destruction of the embryo is morally unacceptable, could one benefit from treatments developed from that source? Or could a scientist, who shares the moral conviction of the Catholic tradition on embryo destruction, be involved in research on cells or lines derived from that source? Could one argue that, since the destruction of the embryo was carried out by others, one's subsequent involvement with the 'fruits' of this initial act, as a scientist or recipient, is morally benign?

Given that we live in an imperfect and sinful world, the issue of our coming into contact with the wrongdoing of others is as old as life itself. Everyday life generates a host of examples: working in a hospital (as a doctor, orderly, electrician) that provides abortion; having business and diplomatic links to a corrupt regime; the amalgamation of Catholic healthcare institutions with other institutions that provide services that are contrary to a Catholic ethos; voting for a political party with a 'mixed' manifesto, and so on. Church teaching and moral theology has responded to this reality using the important, but complex, principle of cooperation and scandal.[19] This moral principle has been applied in recent years to, among other things, the amalgamation of Catholic and non-Catholic institutions and to aspects of the contemporary struggle against HIV.[20]

As part of their initial reflection on this principle, authors often highlighted the different levels of possible cooperation in the wrongdoing of others by drawing upon three examples: the accomplice, the hostage and the taxpayer. Each of these scenarios reveal, in an instructive way, important dimensions of the moral dilemma: *intention, freedom* and *distance* from the immoral act. The accomplice shares the *intention* of the principal wrongdoer, the *freedom* of the hostage is seriously compromised and the taxpayer's involvement in immoral actions (for example, State-funded euthanasia) is remote. The theological tradition continued its analysis by distinguishing, in the first place, between *formal* and *material* cooperation. Formal cooperation is where one approves of the action of the wrongdoer and is, clearly, always wrong. Formal cooperation can be either explicit ('I agree with the actions of the wrongdoer') or implicit. Implicit formal cooperation is 'attributed when, even though the co-operator denies intending the wrongdoer's object, no other explanation can distinguish the co-operator's object from the wrongdoer's object.'[21]

Material cooperation involves associating with the immoral act of another person without approving their action. Obviously there are many different ways in which we can cooperate. Moralists identified different levels of material cooperation: immediate, mediate, proximate, remote, necessary and contingent. Immediate material cooperation occurs when the object of the moral act of the cooperator is indistinguishable from that of the principal agent. This is equivalent to implicit formal cooperation and is, therefore, an unacceptable level of cooperation. Mediate material cooperation, in contrast, occurs when the moral object of the cooperator's act is not that of the wrongdoer. The categories and distinctions of proximate, remote, necessary and contingent were then used to measure the 'quality' of the cooperating act and its 'distance' from the immoral act. The application of these categories to complex situations involves a prudential judgement after taking into account all the relevant information.

The basic thrust of the principle of cooperation and scandal is that we should avoid cooperating in the immoral acts of others; any involvement on our part needs justification and the closer the cooperating act is to the immoral act, the greater the need for justification. Central to this principle was the desire to avoid causing moral confusion and scandal. The *Catechism* defines scandal as 'an attitude or behaviour which leads another to do evil'.[22] There is an acknowledgement here that through our actions we can cause uncertainty in people's minds about the morality of a particular action or cause them to become involved in immoral actions.

Though sometimes difficult in its application, the principle of cooperation and scandal has a distinguished place in the history of moral theology and was used widely in the area of medical ethics. In essence, it addresses the question of *moral consistency* and *moral credibility*. It alerts us to the fact that moral consistency demands that we, as far as possible, disassociate ourselves from cooperating with or enjoying the fruits of an action we judge to be immoral. The action of the Dunnes Stores workers in the 1980s is a good example of the working of the principle. Their stance was that the institution of apartheid was immoral and that moral consistency demanded that they separate themselves from that institution. By refusing to handle goods from South Africa they gave a clear message about their own personal moral stance and helped to undermine that institution by denying it credibility in the public domain. Later the breaking of sporting links to South Africa by the international community was motivated by the same desire to show moral consistency. Receiving stolen goods, on the other hand, serves as an instructive negative example of the principle. We cannot credibly say we believe stealing is a morally bad act while at the same time buying goods stolen by someone else. Even a superficial analysis reveals that our action has the consequence of encouraging thieves in their way of life and contributing to an ethos that sees stealing as morally indifferent. Furthermore, our actions could sow confusion and doubt in the minds of those observing us about the morality of stealing *per se* and about our personal moral stance.

With the production of stem cell lines from embryo destruction, at least three different kinds of cooperation are possible: the cooperation of the State in providing funding, the cooperation of scientists and the cooperation of those who will benefit by receiving tissue, blood, etc. from this source.[23]

In the case of the scientist and the recipient, could one not argue, as many do, that to use or benefit from embryonic stem cells does not necessarily imply approval of embryo destruction? It is, rather, a sensible use of what is commercially and medically available. There are several features about embryonic stem cell research and use that lead inevitably, in my judgement, to the rejection of this approach. Firstly, embryos are deliberately created and destroyed to secure stem cells and other research goals. From the vision of the Catholic moral tradition, the source of the stem cells is morally significant and can't be ignored. This source is morally tainted and the fruit of that source, like stolen goods, should be avoided. It is also relevant that the practice of embryo destruction is supported by a philosophy that sees the pre-implanted embryo as disposable tissue that can be used to bring benefit to others. Cooperating with this practice could credibly be seen as condoning and encouraging this philosophy. The past two decades have witnessed a progressive erosion of respect for the embryo. We have gone rapidly from embryo freezing to experimentation to cloning. Cooperating with such destructive procedures can only encourage the viewing of the embryo as an entity that is devoid of intrinsic value. In this worldview, the embryo acquires significance only through being wanted or useful. This development, surely, has to be contrary to the stance of someone who views the embryo as possessing an inalienable dignity. Successfully treating people from this source could also bestow on embryo destruction a life-saving aura, which could, paradoxically, further contribute to a culture where the embryo is seen as a means to an end. On the other hand, the refusal on the part of scientists and others to work on embryonic stem cell lines or to benefit from treatments developed from that source could help challenge and renew contemporary culture by raising its awareness of the issues involved. Such actions would be both morally consistent and truly prophetic.

The question of cooperation with the culture and practice of embryo destruction has been addressed in recent Church teaching. The American Catholic bishops, for example, have used the language of proximate material cooperation in their condemnation of State funding for embryo destruction.[24] The Pontifical Academy for Life, similarly, argued that the use by scientists of embryonic stem cells, and the differentiated cells obtained from them, supplied by other researchers entails an unacceptable 'proximate material cooperation' in an immoral process.[25]

The Congregation for the Doctrine of the Faith urged scientists to refrain from working with 'biological material' from morally illicit sources, 'in order not to give the impression of a certain toleration or tacit acceptance of actions that are gravely unjust. Any appearance of acceptance would in fact contribute to the growing indifference to, if not the approval of, such actions in certain medical and political circles.'[26]

Benefiting from procedures or treatments linked to the destruction of embryos has also been the subject of some moral analysis in recent Church teaching. *Dignitas personae* acknowledges that individuals could for grave reasons and in exceptional circumstances only avail of treatments or vaccines derived from morally tainted sources.[27] In these exceptional circumstances, people of faith should, however, 'make known their disagreement and ask that their healthcare system make other types of vaccines available.'[28]

When using treatments from illicit sources, in these exceptional circumstances, people should witness clearly to the Catholic moral tradition on the inviolability of human life. The English Catholic bishops, in 1994, adopted a similar position to *Dignitas personae* with regard to the use of a vaccine for rubella, which had been developed from an aborted foetus.[29] In their reflections on the issue, the bishops took into account, in the first place, the fact that the foetus was not aborted in order to develop the vaccine; the decision to have an abortion was, in that particular case, taken for independent reasons. Secondly, they argued that it was a once-off occurrence; the ongoing production of the vaccine did not require any further abortions since the cultured cells reproduced themselves. Thirdly, the taking of the vaccine had substantial benefits for the individual child and for society as a whole. Finally, the fact that the vaccine was the only one available featured centrally in their moral reflection. In conclusion they argued that, though the source of the vaccine was morally problematic, parents were free to give the vaccine to their children.[30]

The English case and the reflections of the English bishops are important because they enable us to identify the similarities and differences between it and the production of embryonic stem cells. A significant, and maybe morally decisive, difference between the rubella case and the production of embryonic stem cells is the *ongoing* nature of embryo destruction in the latter case. The availability of stem cells from other non-controversial sources also marks a decisive difference between these cases. From the perspective of the Catholic moral tradition, the case for benefiting from treatments from this source seems, at best, weak. By benefiting from stem cell treatment from this source, are we inevitably encouraging the practice and its supporting philosophy? By declining such treatments are we, more positively, giving prophetic witness to the value of life?

In conclusion, then, the production and use of embryonic stem cells raises very significant moral issues for individuals and society. Most immediately it raises questions about the status or value of human life during the first few days of its existence. The Catholic moral tradition holds very firmly that human life has a right to be protected from harm from the very beginning of its existence. Secondly, the practice of embryonic stem cell production and use raises questions about how we decide on the goodness of human actions. Are (good) consequences, like the health of individuals or the human family, sufficient to determine the morality of human actions? The Catholic moral tradition has consistently deemed such an approach to morality inadequate. It proposes instead that an adequate evaluation of human actions can only be achieved by taking into account the object of the action, the intention of the acting person and the circumstances within which the action takes place. It is true, also, that embryonic stem cell production and use raises serious questions about the instrumentalisation of human life. The process of using surplus embryos or specifically creating embryos is driven by a philosophy that treats the embryo as a means to an end.

Finally, the existence of non-controversial sources of (adult) stem cells must feature in the process of moral evaluation. Stem cells can be retrieved from sources such as bone marrow, umbilical cord and amniotic fluid. These are promoted by many scientists as realistic alternatives to the use of embryonic stem cells. The conversion of adult cells into induced pluripotent stem cells (iPSC) is now also a reality. This development enables adult cells to be 'reprogrammed' and return to their earlier existence as stem cells. Once consent has been secured, the use of stem cells from these sources does not pose any ethical issues.

To summarise, the approach and conclusions of Church teaching with regard to embryonic stem cell production and use are rooted in Scripture (respect for life), reason (what science tells us about the human embryo) and tradition (the consistent teaching of the Church).

DISCUSSION QUESTIONS
1. Embryonic stem cell research 'advances through the suppression of human lives that are equal in dignity to the lives of other human individuals and to the lives of the researchers themselves' (*Dignitas personae*, paragraph 32). What is the basis of the Church's claim that all human lives are equal in dignity?
2. How important is the goal or 'end' of human well-being?
3. 'It is contradictory to insist that future generations respect the natural environment when our educational systems and laws do not help them to respect themselves.

The book of nature is one and indivisible: it takes in not only the environment but also life, sexuality, marriage, the family, social relations' (*Caritas in veritate*, paragraph 51). What is the link between human ecology and environmental ecology?
4. Should society encourage research with adult stem cells rather than embryonic stem cells?

FURTHER READING

Congregation for the Doctrine of the Faith, *Dignitas personae*, Veritas, 2009, part three.

Corkery, Pádraig, 'Reproductive Technologies: An Irish Contribution to an International Debate', *The Furrow*, 56 (2005), pp. 353–357.

––––, 'The Use of Embryonic Stem Cells: Recent Developments,' *The Furrow*, 53 (2002), pp. 24–34.

Pontifical Academy for Life, *Declaration on the Production and the Scientific and Therapeutic Use of Human Embryonic Stem Cells*, Catholic Truth Society, 2000.

The Irish Council for Bioethics, *Ethical, Scientific and Legal Issues Concerning Stem Cell Research: Opinion*, 2008.

Walter, James J., and Thomas A. Shannon, *Contemporary Issues in Bioethics: A Catholic Perspective*, Rowman & Littlefield Publishers, 2005, chapter 6.

NOTES

1. Congregation for the Doctrine of the Faith, *Dignitas personae*, paragraph 28, gives the following definition: 'Human cloning refers to the asexual or agametic reproduction of the entire human organism in order to produce one or more "copies" which, from a genetic perspective, are substantially identical to the single original.'
2. Pontifical Academy for Life, *Declaration on the Production and the Scientific and Therapeutic Use of Human Embryonic Stem Cells*, Catholic Truth Society, 2000, p. 9.
3. *Report of the Commission on Assisted Human Reproduction*, xvi.

4. Ibid., xvii.
5. Ibid., xviii.
6. The Irish Council for Bioethics, *Ethical, Scientific and Legal Issues Concerning Stem Cell Research: Opinion*, 2008.
7. Ibid., paragraph 41.
8. Ibid., paragraph 44.
9. Ibid., paragraph 45.
10. Ibid.
11. Ibid., paragraph 46.
12. Ibid.
13. Ibid., paragraph 54.
14. Ibid.
15. Ibid. Emphasis mine.
16. Ibid., paragraph 56.
17. Ibid., paragraph 59.
18. Congregation for the Doctrine of the Faith, *Dignitas personae*, paragraphs 28–30, 33; Pontifical Academy for Life, *Declaration on the Production and the Scientific and Therapeutic Use of Human Embryonic Stem Cells*, Catholic Truth Society, 2000, p. 10.
19. Congregation for the Doctrine of the Faith, *Dignitas personae*, paragraphs 34–36; Helen Watt (ed.), *Cooperation, Complicity & Conscience*, Linacre Centre, 2005; Helen Watt, *Life and Death in Healthcare Ethics*, Routledge, 2000, chapter 6; Thomas O'Donnell, *Medicine and Christian Morality*, Third Edition, Alba House, 1996, pp. 34–48.
20. James F. Keenan (ed.), *Catholic Ethicists on HIV/AIDS Prevention*, Continuum, 2000, section 5: 'Using the Principle of Co-operation', pp. 177–211; Kieran Cronin, 'Harm Reduction and Drug Use', *The Furrow*, 52 (2001), pp. 154–163.
21. United States Conference of Catholic Bishops, 'Ethical and Religious Directives for Catholic Health Care Services', *Origins*, 24 (15 December 1994), pp. 449–461, 'Appendix'. See also paragraph 69. Later editions of these Directives omitted the 'Appendix' with its definition of the principle and its various terms.
22. *Catechism of the Catholic Church*, paragraph 2284.
23. See Pádraig Corkery, 'The Use of Embryonic Stem Cells: Recent Developments', *The Furrow*, 53 (2002), pp. 24–34, 29.

24. See, for example, the statements of a range of American bishops concerning the provision of federal funding in *Origins*, 31 (30 August 2001), pp. 205–212.
25. Pontifical Academy for Life, *Declaration on the Production and the Scientific and Therapeutic Use of Human Embryonic Stem Cells*, Catholic Truth Society, 2000, p. 10.
26. Congregation for the Doctrine of the Faith, *Dignitas personae*, paragraph 35.
27. Ibid.
28. Ibid.
29. Pádraig Corkery, 'The Use of Embryonic Stem Cells: Recent Developments', *The Furrow*, 53 (2002), pp. 24–34, p. 31.
30. Ibid., p. 32.

4   Ethical Issues at the End of Life

OVER RECENT DECADES, THE ABILITY OF MEDICINE TO sustain human life has grown enormously. With a new range of skills and technology doctors can intervene, even in the most difficult of circumstances, to save a person's life. We are all aware of persons and families who have benefited from the awesome skills of modern physicians and the latest advances in medical science.

Occasionally, however, medical practitioners can prevent death but are unable to restore consciousness or health. Patients are left in a state of limbo; alive but attached to artificial life-sustaining interventions with no hope of recovery. In these circumstances, people rightly question the extent of our obligation to sustain human life. Individuals wonder whether human life is to be preserved at all costs and whether we are obliged to use all the treatments and interventions at our disposal to keep people alive?

This is not, of course, a new question. Ethicists and the books of medical ethics pondered on this question long before modern advances in medical science. But the question is asked with a greater urgency today and is debated more openly in public debates, civil courts and academic works. A range of interesting questions need to be engaged if we accept that we are not obliged to use every kind of medical intervention to keep people alive. What criteria do we use to justify the withdrawal or withholding of life-sustaining interventions? Who should be involved in that decision-making? Is there a significant difference between the death of a person through omission and commission? How does euthanasia differ from the withdrawal of life-sustaining interventions?

Answering these questions has caused much debate and disagreement in many societies in recent years. Court cases concerning the care of Karen Quinlan (USA), Tony Bland (England), Ward of Court (Ireland) and Terri Schiavo (USA) received extensive coverage in the media and in public debate. These cases raised important questions for the individuals and families involved, as well as for society and for healthcare professionals.

The Response of the Catholic Moral Tradition

The Catholic moral tradition has approached the question of our obligation to sustain human life from within the Christian worldview that shapes and directs its response to issues in the domain of healthcare and elsewhere. Three aspects of this vision in particular direct its approach and shape its conclusions in this area. Firstly, there is an acceptance of the naturalness of death. The Christian self-understanding accepts that we are mortal beings for whom death is a part of life; it is an essential and inescapable part of who we are. Secondly, the Christian community experiences human life as a gift from God that should be embraced with gratitude and reverence. As stewards of the gift of life, we have a duty to protect and respect our own life and the lives of others. Finally, the claim of Christian anthropology that we are created in the image of God plays a decisive role in constructing the Catholic tradition's response to this issue.

An immediate consequence of this way of understanding the human person is the belief that we are more than one-dimensional. There is a spiritual dimension to our lives that needs to be acknowledged and affirmed. In this Christian self-understanding, God is experienced as our origin and our destiny; we come from God and return to God. This perspective is made explicit in Christ's resurrection. For believers, death is engaged through the eyes of a resurrection faith and is experienced, consequently, not as an end, but as the beginning of a new life with God. Since Christ rose from the dead, believers confidently hope to share in the same destiny. This faith is clearly and prayerfully articulated in the Preface for the Dead: 'Lord, for your faithful people life is changed not ended. When our mortal bodies lie in death we gain an everlasting dwelling place in heaven.'

These perspectives give us a very particular starting point when we approach the question of our obligation to sustain human life; death is a part of our nature, but has been ultimately defeated by the resurrection of Christ. The reality of our own mortality and the mortality of our loved ones is processed through the prism of Christian hope. Sadness, pain and a profound sense of loss still accompany the experience of death, but are mediated through the lens of a resurrection faith.

Working out of this framework, the theological tradition proposes that we are obliged to use only 'ordinary' treatments to keep people alive. These treatments are deemed morally obligatory. 'Extraordinary' treatments may be used but are morally optional. This language of 'ordinary' and 'extraordinary' treatments does, of course, beg the question of how to decide which treatments are 'ordinary' and 'extraordinary'. Is there a list of such treatments available for us to consult when engaged in the process of decision-making?

A widely used and authoritative textbook of medical ethics defined the terms as follows:

> Ordinary means of preserving life are all medicines, treatments and operations, which offer a reasonable hope of benefit for the patient and which can be obtained and used without excessive expense, pain, or other inconvenience.[1]

The author understood extraordinary means of preserving life as:

> All medicines, treatments, and operations, which cannot be obtained or used without excessive expense, pain, or other inconvenience, or which, if used, would not offer a reasonable hope of benefit.[2]

Working with these definitions, the theological community proposed two criteria, *benefit* and *burden*, to assist in determining whether care was ordinary (morally obligatory) or extraordinary (morally optional). In this framework, the criterion of benefit is almost transparent while that of burden is more opaque. In general, the latter criterion was understood in terms of the physical, financial and psychological impact of the intervention on the patient and his or her family.[3]

This was the standard theological framework that appeared in textbooks of medical ethics and which informed the ethos and practice in Catholic hospitals worldwide. It has an important place in the history of medical ethics and has ongoing relevance in a changed and changing world. Its strength is that it provides us with a useful framework and set of criteria that enable us to approach complicated human dilemmas. It is a person-centred approach that recognises the uniqueness of each person and each set of circumstances. It recognises that what may be 'ordinary' for one person, and hence morally obligatory, could be 'extraordinary' and, therefore, morally optional for another because of their differing circumstances. It is a framework that must be applied to a particular person in a *particular* set of circumstances. The application of this framework to a *particular* person involves prudential judgements after all the relevant information has been considered. It is possible that reasonable people may differ in their assessment of the relevant information and in their judgement concerning what is 'ordinary' or 'extraordinary'.

Today the terms 'proportionate' and 'disproportionate' medicine are sometimes used to describe the same insight and framework. We are not obliged to use every intervention at our disposal to keep people alive, but only those that are *proportionate* – those medical interventions that offer the person a reasonable hope of benefit without imposing too severe a burden.

It might be instructive at this stage to look at how the Magisterium has used this framework as it responded to questions about the care of the sick and dying. In an often-quoted address to doctors in 1957, Pope Pius XII had this to say:

> But normally one is held to use only ordinary means – according to circumstances of persons, places, times and cultures – that is to say, means that do not involve any grave burden for oneself or another. A more strict obligation would be too burdensome for most people and would render the attainment of the higher, more important good too difficult. Life, health, all temporal activities are in fact subordinated to spiritual ends.[4]

The person-centred and circumstance-sensitive nature of the framework is evident in the early part of the statement. Medical interventions cannot be classified 'ordinary' or 'extraordinary' in the abstract. This categorising can only be done after all the circumstances have been taken into account. The last line of this intervention is also worth reflecting on. It sums up very sharply a central insight of the Christian faith. The meaning of our earthly existence is not to be found in mere physical existence, but in terms of our relationship with God and others. Physical life is to be valued and protected, but it is not the ultimate value. There are realities and experiences that are more important than physical existence. It is this truth that enables people to love others selflessly and at great cost to themselves in terms of health, energy or comfort. This truth also inspired many to give their lives in the service of others or to be martyred for their Christian faith.

In 1980, the Congregation for the Doctrine of the Faith issued a significant letter on the issue of euthanasia.[5] The immediate context was the public discussion on the content of the civil law on euthanasia. Many societies were at that time contemplating a change in the prohibition on euthanasia. In the course of its response to this discussion, the Congregation clarified the Church's approach to the withdrawing or withholding of life-saving interventions and how these actions differed from euthanasia:

> Everyone has the duty to care for his/her health. ... However, is it necessary in all circumstances to have recourse to all possible remedies? In the past moralists replied that one is never obliged to use 'extraordinary' means. This reply, which as a principle still holds good, is perhaps less clear today, by reason of the imprecision of the term and the rapid progress made in the treatment of sickness.[6]

The validity of the theological tradition's framework of 'ordinary' and 'extraordinary' treatments is affirmed by the Congregation while, at the same time, acknowledging that the complexity of modern healthcare makes it more difficult to determine exactly what these terms mean. The document proceeds, however, to outline steps to assist in the 'unpacking' of these terms:

> [S]tudying the type of treatment to be used, its degree of complexity or risk, its cost and the possibilities of using it, and comparing these elements with the result that can be expected, taking into account the state of the sick person and his/her physical and moral resources.[7]

The last line of the quotation highlights again the person-centred nature of the theological approach. There is a clear acceptance that people may differ in both physical and moral resources. The reality and implications of differing physical resources are self-evident, while the concept of moral resources needs a word of clarification. What exactly did the Congregation have in mind when they introduced the concept of *moral resources*? We must assume that the virtues – including patience, courage, perseverance and hope – would be included here. It is also true that individuals may be more or less prepared for death. Some may be at peace with the prospect of dying while others, in similar circumstances, may be afraid or need more time to be reconciled to God and family. There cannot, therefore, be a 'one size fits all' approach when it comes to making decisions in this area of life.

The document goes on to clarify that the refusal of 'extraordinary' care is not the equivalent of suicide but 'should be considered as an acceptance of the human condition, or a wish to avoid the application of a medical procedure disproportionate to the results that can be expected, or a desire not to impose excessive expense on the family or the community.'[8]

The *Catechism of the Catholic Church*, published in 1992, dealt briefly with this subject in its treatment of the fifth commandment:

> Discontinuing medical procedures that are burdensome, dangerous, extraordinary, or disproportionate to the expected outcome can be legitimate; it is the refusal of 'over zealous' treatment. Here one does not will to cause death; one's inability to impede it is merely accepted.[9]

In this passage, we note that the *Catechism*, while articulating the traditional language of 'extraordinary', 'burden' and 'disproportionate', does not indicate how these terms, and others, can be unpacked.

Finally, *Evangelium vitae*, published in 1995, clearly highlighted the legitimacy of refusing 'extraordinary' or 'disproportionate' treatments, while at the same time condemning euthanasia:

> It needs to be determined whether the means of treatment available are objectively proportionate to the prospects for improvement. To forego extraordinary or disproportionate means is not the equivalent of suicide or euthanasia; it rather expresses acceptance of the human condition in the face of death.[10]

To summarise, then, the Catholic moral tradition holds that we are not obliged to use all our resources to sustain human life. Though the tradition promotes the principle of the sacredness of human life, it does not see the preservation of life as an absolute. This approach is shaped by a belief in the naturalness of death, a Christian anthropology and Christian hope. We are obliged to use only means that carry some reasonable hope of benefit and don't impose too great a burden on the person and his/her family. The criterion of burden was understood in terms of pain, expense and psychological health. Ideally, the person themselves should be involved in this decision-making, since only they can truly evaluate their physical and moral resources. When this is not possible, because of physical or mental debility, the decision should be made by the family of the patient, in consultation with medical advice. Because the determination of what constitutes 'ordinary' and 'extraordinary' care involves prudential judgements, it is occasionally possible that reasonable people may differ in their judgements about the care of a particular person.

The Catholic moral tradition's approach to this important and complex area of healthcare has been the subject of significant misunderstanding and, consequently, criticism in public discussion over recent decades. Since the withdrawal of life-sustaining treatments results in the death of a person, some argue that this act is, in fact, an act of 'passive' euthanasia. They would, consequently, contend that the Church in its very vocal opposition to active euthanasia is being inconsistent and hypocritical. Opponents of the Church's stance, in their (mis)understanding, argue that because the Church allows 'passive' euthanasia, it should also allow 'active' euthanasia, since both result in a death that is foreseen. This misunderstanding of the Church's stance on euthanasia and on the difference between euthanasia and the withdrawal of 'extraordinary' treatments is one that needs a careful response.

The term euthanasia is derived from two Greek words, *'eu'* and *'thanatos'*, which literally mean a 'good' or 'easy death'. In everyday parlance, euthanasia is most often understood as 'mercy killing'. There is a range of terms used today to describe various types of euthanasia. 'Active' euthanasia describes a situation where the death of a person is intentionally caused through some active intervention. 'Passive' euthanasia occurs when one intentionally causes the death of someone by withdrawing or withholding some treatment or intervention that the person is entitled to. 'Voluntary' euthanasia implies that the person, with full knowledge of the consequences of their decision, has requested euthanasia. 'Involuntary' euthanasia describes the scenario where euthanasia is carried out on a person against their clear and expressed wishes. 'Non-voluntary' euthanasia occurs where euthanasia is carried out on those who are incapable of giving or denying consent because of their mental or physical incapacity.

The contemporary debate on euthanasia, in England and other countries of the European Union, concerns the legalisation of voluntary euthanasia, both 'active' and 'passive'. In the United States, on the other hand, the debate has focused largely on the availability of physician-assisted suicide. In the State of Oregon, for example, physicians can make available a lethal cocktail, which the patient him/herself administers. In this scenario, physicians enable patients to end their own lives.

Arguments in favour of voluntary euthanasia in society are generally built on the principle of autonomy and the right to self-determination. Human freedom, it is argued, is a fundamental dimension and demand of our existence. It is through the exercise of our freedom that we give direction and shape to our lives. Through the exercise of our freedom, we determine the kind of person we want to be and the kind of lives we want to lead. We freely make decisions that determine some of the most important aspects of our lives, including our marital status or vocation in life. We should also, it is argued, be allowed to determine the time and circumstances of our death since our death is inevitable. The ultimate act of self-determination would be to choose the time and circumstances of our demise.

A secondary argument advanced in favour of euthanasia draws upon a standard principle used in bioethics, the principle of benevolence, which directs us towards doing good for others. We honour this principle, it is argued, when we respond to the free and fully-informed request of an individual for euthanasia in order to relieve them of a level of pain that they experience as overwhelming.

How does the Catholic moral tradition respond to the arguments supporting the call to legalise euthanasia? The first major Church document on euthanasia provides a very helpful definition that clearly identifies key distinctions:

> By euthanasia is understood an action or an omission which of itself or by intention causes death, in order that all suffering may in this way be eliminated. Euthanasia's terms of reference, therefore, are to be found in the intention of the will and in the methods used.[11]

From the perspective of moral reflection and moral clarity, the important point of this definition is that euthanasia involves *intentionally causing* the death of another, by omission or commission, in order to lessen their suffering. In this way it differs fundamentally from the withdrawing or withholding of 'extraordinary' treatment. In the latter scenario, the intention is not to kill the patient but to relieve him/her of an intervention that is overly burdensome or hopeless. The death of the person is not intended but accepted with regret. It is not, therefore, euthanasia, 'passive' or otherwise, because there is no intention to cause the death of another.

The Church's teaching on euthanasia is clear and consistent. It judges it to be 'a violation of the divine law, an offence against the dignity of the human person, a crime against life, and an attack on humanity'.[12] The Christian tradition holds that the direct taking of the life of an innocent person is contrary to the moral law. They root their argument both in natural law and Revelation. Reasoned reflection on life identifies human life as a core value. Consequently, the protection and valuing of human life has been central to the ethos of all societies. Valuing human life and protecting it from direct attack is the foundation on which societies are built. Scripture and, particularly, the ethos of the New Testament prohibit the taking of innocent human life. In the vision of Scripture, life is seen as a gift from God and God alone has sovereignty over life. Furthermore, human stewardship calls us to be responsible stewards of the great gift of life.

In conclusion, then, the Church teaches that euthanasia is 'a grave violation of the law of God, since it is the deliberate and morally unacceptable killing of a human person.'[13] It bases its moral stance on the three moral sources identified in chapter one: 'The natural law and upon the written Word of God … the Church's Tradition and … the ordinary and universal Magisterium'.[14] Rather than seeing euthanasia as a mercy killing, it sees it as a 'false mercy, and indeed a disturbing "perversion" of mercy'.[15]

Discussion Questions
1. Why does the Catholic Tradition allow for the withdrawal or withholding of 'extraordinary' treatments?
2. By withdrawing life-support systems, are we 'playing God' and, therefore, going beyond our nature as 'creatures'?
3. How does euthanasia differ from withdrawing 'extraordinary' or 'disproportionate' treatments?

4. What did *Evangelium vitae* mean by describing euthanasia as 'a false mercy, and indeed a "perversion" of mercy'?

FURTHER READING

Congregation for the Doctrine of the Faith, *Declaration on Euthanasia*, 1980.

Leies, John A. et. al, *Handbook on Critical Life Issues*, Third Edition, The National Catholic Bioethics Centre, 2004, Part III.

O'Rourke, Kevin (ed.), *A Primer for Healthcare Ethics*, Second Edition, Georgetown University Press, 2000, part three.

Watt, Helen, *Life and Death in Healthcare Ethics*, Routledge, 2000, chapter 1.

NOTES

1. Gerard Kelly SJ, *Medico Moral Problems*, Clonmore & Reynolds, 1960, p. 129.
2. Ibid.
3. Ibid., p. 132: 'Yet he need not spend money or incur a debt which would impose a very great hardship on himself or his family, because this kind of hardship would be more than a "reasonable" or "moderate" care of health and therefore more than God would ordinarily demand.'
4. Pope Pius XII, 'The Prolongation of Life', *The Pope Speaks*, 4.4 (Spring 1958), pp. 395–398.
5. Congregation for the Doctrine of the Faith, *Euthanasia*, 1980.
6. Ibid., section IV.
7. Ibid.
8. Ibid.
9. *Catechism of the Catholic Church*, Veritas, 1995, paragraph 2278.
10. *Evangelium vitae*, Veritas, 1995, paragraph 65.
11. Congregation for the Doctrine of the Faith, *Euthanasia*, 1980, section 2.
12. Ibid.
13. *Evangelium vitae*, paragraph 65.
14. Ibid.
15. Ibid., paragraph 66.

5 The Administration of Nutrition and Hydration to Persons in a Permanent Vegetative State (PVS)

THE FRAMEWORK FOR DISCUSSING THE CARE OF THE seriously ill, outlined in the last chapter, is still valid and well utilised in Catholic healthcare facilities across the globe. However, in recent decades it has had to engage with a new situation of care that has tested its coherence and credibility. The case in point is that of the person in a permanent vegetative state (PVS). Persons in such a condition are permanently unconscious, but their hearts are beating and they are breathing on their own. They are not, therefore, assisted or maintained by any mechanical intervention. They are sustained in this condition by the provision of nutrition and hydration through artificial means. Because of the excellence of contemporary healthcare, persons can live in this condition for over twenty years. In light of this fact, many people question whether the provision of nutrition and hydration to such persons is ethically justified.

The most recent case of this kind to be debated in the public domain was that of Terri Schiavo. Her case generated a great deal of discussion and disagreement amongst commentators from the worlds of ethics, law and medicine. The central question debated was whether the continued provision of such care was 'ordinary' and, therefore, morally obligatory, or 'extraordinary' and, therefore, morally optional.

Some argued that the provision of such care should be viewed as a form of patient abuse through overtreatment. Others suggested that the denial of such care was an example of patient neglect.

This debate on the appropriate level of care for persons in a PVS has been conducted within Church, legal and medical circles for the past twenty years. Over the course of those years, the principal areas of agreement and conflict have been identified. It is instructive, I think, to identify these central points of the debate before considering recent Catholic teaching on the matter. From the academic and pastoral literature generated over many years, it is possible to identify at least five areas of disagreement.

(1) THE NATURE OF NUTRITION AND HYDRATION
The first source of disagreement focuses on the nature of artificially administered nutrition and hydration. Is the provision of such nutrition and hydration to be considered a basic human care that everyone is entitled to, or, alternatively, is it to be deemed a medical treatment that can be withdrawn if it is deemed futile or without benefit? In the early years of the debate, for example, the English Catholic bishops, while they were clear that it was unacceptable to remove nutrition/hydration with the *intention* of causing death, were uncertain as to whether the provision of nutrition/hydration was a medical treatment or a basic care.[1]

Commentators, in general, have approached this question from two different perspectives. The first group argue that the provision of nutrition/hydration is a basic care or first-order human response, which we are obliged to give to everyone. In the Ward of Court case, for example, the Irish Medical Council and An Bord Altranais adopted this approach.[2] The obligation to provide such care was compared to the obligation to keep patients warm and clean. Some commentators also argued that food and drink are symbolically rich since we welcome people into the human family by providing food and drink. To deny this to anyone, and especially the most vulnerable, they argued, is a step backwards for humanity. Furthermore, some commentators utilised the slippery-slope argument that if we deny nutrition and hydration, even to a limited and well-defined group of persons like those in a PVS, such a practice will inevitably be extended to include other categories of patients that are vulnerable and have a poor quality of life.

The other side of the argument maintained that when nutrition and hydration is administered artificially it should be classified as a medical treatment. Like all other medical treatments, it can be withdrawn or withheld if it is judged to be futile or too burdensome. This stance was reflected, for example, in the judgement of the High Court in the Tony Bland case.

(2) What Happens When the Nutrition/Hydration is Removed?

The second point of disagreement centred on how commentators understood the consequences of the removal of nutrition/hydration. Does the removal of the nutrition/hydration *cause* the death of the patient or simply *allow* the patient to die? Those who adopted the latter approach argued that the patient-person already had a fatal pathology and that the withdrawal of the nutrition/hydration simply allowed that fatal pathology to take its natural course. This stance was adopted by the Texan bishops in the early part of the debate within the Catholic community.[3] Those who adopted the former approach argued that the patient died, not because he/she was in a PVS, but because of a new set of circumstances – starvation and dehydration – that were intentionally and knowingly introduced. In other words, the death of Tony Bland and others was directly intended and caused by those who removed their feeding.

(3) What are the Benefits of Nutrition/Hydration?
The criterion of *benefit* is a standard part of the traditional 'ordinary'/'extraordinary' approach to medical care. The case of a person in a PVS raises, in a new and dramatic way, questions about how we measure or understand benefit. What benefits does the provision of nutrition/hydration confer on the patient in this case? Some argue that continued physical existence is a benefit and, therefore, the provision of nutrition/hydration, which enables the person to stay alive, must be deemed to be beneficial. Others approach the debate quite differently. They argue that *benefit* must be measured against some understanding of the goals of life. The first step in this approach is to try and clarify what the purpose or goal of human existence is. Once this has been identified, questions can then be asked about the continued provision of nutrition/hydration. Does the provision of such care enable the goal of life to be achieved?

(4) Dying or Seriously Ill?
The fourth source of disagreement centred on how to classify persons in a PVS: are they dying or seriously ill? In the courts, in the Tony Bland and Terri Schiavo cases, for example, there was disagreement amongst medical experts on this point.

(5) Who Decides?
Finally, commentators disagreed on the role that family and the courts should be assigned given that the PVS person cannot decide for him/herself. If there is no indication of the person's wishes, in a 'Living Will' or otherwise, who should

make decisions about their care? Should those decisions be made by the families involved, by the healthcare team in consultation with the families or by the courts?

These points of disagreement, evident in the contributions of ethicians and other experts, were also reflected in the Catholic theological community during the early years of the debate. During the debate on Tony Bland, as noted earlier, the English bishops were unsure as to whether nutrition/hydration should be classified as medical treatment or as a basic care. The American Catholic bishops, in their early comments on the moral dilemma, argued that there should be 'a presumption' in favour of providing nutrition/hydration, but that this presumption should yield when such feeding is deemed to 'have no medically reasonable hope of sustaining life or pose excessive risks or burdens'.[4] Theological journals during this time period also reveal a lively debate among Catholic moral theologians as they wrestled with this complex moral issue.[5]

It is also worth noting that both the *Catechism of the Catholic Church* and *Evangelium vitae* did not comment on the moral debate surrounding the care of persons in a PVS, even though this debate was well advanced at the time of their publication. Both documents simply proposed the traditional framework of 'ordinary'/'extraordinary' treatment without applying it to the particular case of persons in a PVS.[6]

It is important to highlight that there were also significant areas of agreement among Catholic moralists during this time as they reflected on this complex human drama. Even though they held conflicting views on the morality of withdrawing nutrition and hydration from persons in a PVS, they were united in their acceptance of the following principles:

1. At the heart of the debate is the question of how best to care for vulnerable persons who are in a PVS. An adequate response must acknowledge, respect and promote the dignity of such persons.

2. All agreed that those in a PVS are persons and must be respected as persons. In this regard many commentators found the term 'vegetative state' regrettable and dangerous. It could be understood in a reductionist way that gives the impression that we are dealing with sub-personal life. Catholic authors consistently argued that those in a PVS are persons with an innate dignity and rights. The central question that needs to be addressed is how best the dignity of persons in a PVS can be respected and promoted.[7]

3. Catholic contributors were also in agreement that it is not morally acceptable to withdraw nutrition/hydration with the *intention* of causing death. Catholic authors who favoured the withdrawal of nutrition/hydration argued that the intention was to relieve the person of an intervention that was burdensome or of no benefit, thus allowing the person to die of their underlying fatal pathology. Their death was, therefore, not intended but permitted.

In March 2004, Pope John Paul II made a significant, if not decisive, contribution to the debate among Catholic theologians and healthcare providers on the care of persons in a PVS. In his address, Pope John Paul II argued that:

> The administration of water and food, even when provided by artificial means, always represents a natural means of preserving life, not a medical act. Its use …

should be considered, in principle, ordinary and proportionate and as such morally obligatory, insofar as and until it is seen to have attained its proper finality, which in the present case consists in providing nourishment to the patient and alleviation of his suffering.[8]

Furthermore, he claimed that since death by starvation or dehydration is the only possible outcome of the withdrawal of feeding, such withdrawal 'ends up becoming, if done knowingly and willingly, true and proper *euthanasia by omission*'.[9]

The content and implications of this intervention are important and worthy of further consideration. In terms of the five areas of disagreement outlined above, it is clear that the Pope took a definite stance on several issues. In the first place, it is clear that he judged that the provision of nutrition and hydration to persons in a PVS is a basic human care and not a medical treatment, which every person is entitled to as a right. Equally, he was clear that the withdrawal of such feeding was the direct cause of the person's death rather than the underlying pathology. Furthermore, in his analysis, the withdrawal of such feeding, if done knowingly and willingly, is euthanasia by omission. He allowed only one exception to the obligation to provide nutrition and hydration to persons in a PVS. This exception arises when the nutrition and hydration cannot be assimilated by the person and cannot, therefore, achieve its goal.

This statement by Pope John Paul II generated a lot of discussion among Catholic moralists.[10] Important questions were raised about the content, status and binding force of his contribution. The impact of the statement can be clearly seen in, amongst others, the contributions made by the Catholic bishops of Florida in the Terri Schiavo case. In a statement issued *before* Pope John Paul's intervention, they argued:

If Mrs Schiavo's feeding tube were to be removed because the nutrition she receives is of no use to her, or because she is near death, or because it is unreasonably burdensome for her, her family, or caregivers, it could be seen as permissible.[11]

Here the bishops identify three circumstances where the use of nutrition/hydration becomes morally optional. The last example of 'unreasonably burdensome' reflects the standard language of moral theology that allows, in practice, for a wide range of circumstances in which withdrawal could be morally appropriate.

In the same statement, they also identified motives that they deemed morally unacceptable:

But if her feeding tube were to be removed to *intentionally* cause her death, or because her life is perceived to be useless, or because it is believed that the quality of her life is such that she would be better off, this would be wrong.[12]

Their statement published *after* the papal intervention reflects the moral analysis and conclusions of that statement and is, therefore, far more restrictive. In their contribution they argued that nutrition/hydration, 'as long as they effectively provide nourishment and help provide comfort', should be seen 'as part of what we owe to all who are helpless and in our care'.[13]

This contribution by Pope John Paul II was expected by many to bring to an end, at least within the Catholic faith community, the debate on the appropriate care of persons in a PVS. However, questions still remained as to the status of the contribution and its binding force. Is the contribution of Pope John Paul II on this issue to be regarded as binding official Church teaching or as his personal contribution to the theological debate? Questions also arose as to the exact meaning and scope of the phrase 'in principle'. Are there other exceptions (other than that of non-assimilation) to the general obligation to always provide nutrition and hydration? Because of these remaining questions and uncertainties, the American Catholic bishops sought clarity from the Congregation of the Doctrine of the Faith in 2007. The two questions submitted by the bishops, and the reply of the Congregation, are short and focused. For that reason, I will present the complete text:[14]

> FIRST QUESTION: Is the administration of food and water (whether by natural or artificial means) to a patient in a 'vegetative state' morally obligatory except when they cannot be assimilated by the patient's body or cannot be administered to the patient without causing significant physical discomfort?
>
> RESPONSE: Yes. The administration of food and water even by artificial means is, in principle, an ordinary and proportionate means of preserving life. It is therefore obligatory to the extent to which, and for as long as, it is shown to accomplish its proper finality, which is the hydration and nourishment of the patient. In this way suffering and death by starvation and dehydration are prevented.
>
> SECOND QUESTION: When nutrition and hydration are being supplied by artificial means to a patient in a 'permanent vegetative state', may they be disconnected when competent physicians judge with moral certainty that the patient will never recover consciousness?

RESPONSE: No. A patient in a 'permanent vegetative state' is a person with fundamental human dignity and must, therefore, receive ordinary and proportionate care which includes, in principle, the administration of water and food even by artificial means.

The position advanced by the CDF was not unexpected in light of the intervention of Pope John Paul II in 2004. The *Responses* appear on first reading to be clear and unambiguous. The administration of food and water, even artificially, is 'normal' treatment and hence morally obligatory, except in the case where the patient is unable to assimilate them. It is worth noting at this stage, however, that the second possible exception raised by the American bishops in question one – when food and water cannot be administered to the patient without causing significant physical discomfort – was not explicitly addressed by the CDF. We must assume that the failure to address this exception was deliberate and not an omission. It is reasonable to conclude, therefore, that this exception is not permitted. The provision of nutrition and hydration is, therefore, morally obligatory in all circumstances other than when such nutrition and hydration cannot 'accomplish its proper finality'.

When issuing the *Responses*, the Congregation for the Doctrine of the Faith also issued a *Commentary*.[15] This text provides some useful clarifications and background information. It is, unfortunately, also the source of some confusion, since it allows for exceptions that go beyond those admitted in the *Responses*. It also employs the criterion of *burden*, which is not used in the *Responses* or in the intervention of Pope John Paul II.

It affirms that the provision of nutrition/hydration is morally obligatory *in principle*. However, it acknowledges three circumstances where such provision is not morally mandated. The first two are not problematic and, indeed, one of them is dealt with in the *Responses*. The first involves circumstances of poverty and underdevelopment where the provision of such nutrition and hydration 'may be physically impossible, and then *ad impossibilia nemo tenetur*'.[16] The second circumstance is already mentioned explicitly in the *Response*. It deals with the situation where 'a patient may be unable to assimilate food and liquids, so that their provision becomes altogether useless'.[17] The third circumstance mentioned is one that introduces the traditional theological language of *burden* and would seem to allow for a range of exceptions that go beyond those identified in the *Responses* and in the contribution of Pope John Paul II. For the sake of accuracy it is important to reproduce the text itself:

> Finally, the possibility is not absolutely excluded that, in rare cases, artificial nourishment and hydration may be excessively burdensome for the patient or may cause significant physical discomfort, for example resulting from complications in the use of the means employed.[18]

There are two distinct exceptions allowed here that go beyond those deemed permissible in the *Response*. The language of burden reflects the traditional language of moral theology as it attempted to measure the impact of a medical intervention on a person. As indicated already, this term has found its way into magisterial teaching, including the *Catechism*. The term does, of course, need to be 'unpacked' and 'measured'. Traditionally, theologians understood burden in broad terms: physical discomfort, psychological and spiritual distress, and financial considerations. It allowed for the possibility that because of differing physical, spiritual, emotional and financial resources, an intervention may be burdensome for one person and not for another in somewhat similar medical circumstances. In the case of those in a PVS, it could allow for an approach that is more open-ended, sensitive and person-centred. Could continued feeding be seen as *excessively burdensome* for someone who, working out of a Christian faith vision, had expressed a desire to be allowed to die peacefully unattached to artificial aids?

The second exception mentioned, *significant physical discomfort*, was raised by the American bishops in their questions, but not explicitly dealt with in the *Responses*. Does its acceptance here indicate a less rigid approach to that proposed in the *Responses*?

The *Commentary*, in my estimation, introduces an element of confusion into the discussion. Though it is not part of the *Responses*, and, therefore, its doctrinal status is uncertain, it was published by the same Congregation and accompanied the former document. On the one hand, it allows for exceptions that go beyond those explicitly approved by the *Responses* and employs the criterion of *burden*, which was noticeably absent from that statement. On the other hand, in its concluding paragraph it contends:

> These exceptional cases, however, take nothing away from the general ethical criterion, according to which the provision of water and food, even by artificial means, always represents a natural means for preserving life, and is not a therapeutic treatment. Its use should therefore be considered ordinary and proportionate, even when the 'vegetative state' is prolonged.[19]

CONCLUSION

The questions submitted by the American bishops for clarification are important. The care of persons in a PVS is a significant pastoral issue for the Church in America and elsewhere. The central challenge is to respond to their plight in a way that is respectful of their dignity as persons. Teasing out the implications of human dignity for persons in a PVS is not an easy task. On the one hand, there are specific actions and attitudes, like treating the person in a PVS as a 'non-person' or intentionally causing their death, that are clearly incompatible with human dignity. On the other hand, questions still remain as to the extent of the obligation to provide nutrition/hydration to those in a PVS. Are we obliged to provide such feeding indefinitely?

The intervention of Pope John Paul II and the *Responses* from the Congregation for the Doctrine of the Faith have made a valuable contribution to this discussion. They are clear and unambiguous on an important question that was disputed by commentators, Catholic and otherwise. The stance of both documents is that, in the case of persons in a PVS, artificially administered nutrition/hydration is a basic human care and not a medical treatment. It is, therefore, morally obligatory. The only exception they recognise is when the nutrition/hydration is unable to achieve its purpose because the person cannot assimilate it. This approach excludes, therefore, considering the burden (psychological, spiritual, financial or physical) that continued feeding may impose on the person or his/her family.

The *Commentary* provided by the CDF affirms the central insights and thrust of Pope John Paul II's intervention and those of the *Responses*. However, in one regard, it deviates significantly from the parameters proposed in those documents and, in this way, highlights an important element of the Catholic moral tradition. By suggesting that feeding could be withdrawn if it was too *burdensome* for the person, it allows for a wide range of considerations to be taken on board. This approach is more open-ended and allows the personality, moral vision and circumstances of the patient to have a significant impact on the final decision. It could be argued that the *Commentary* works out of a broader canvas than that employed by Pope John Paul II in his intervention or that of the Congregation of the Doctrine of the Faith in their *Responses*; a canvas that is more in keeping with the Catholic moral tradition because it more readily accepts that life is not an end in itself.

DISCUSSION QUESTIONS
1. How useful is the 'ordinary'/'extraordinary' framework when discussing the care of persons in a PVS?
2. Why is the language of 'vegetative state' not the 'most felicitous when applied to human beings' (Pope John Paul II)?
3. What are the 'benefits' that accrue from the continued administration of nutrition and hydration to persons in a PVS?

FURTHER READING
Caplan, Arthur L. et. al (eds), *The Case of Terri Schiavo*, Prometheus Books, 2006.
Corkery, Pádraig, 'Beyond the Terri Schiavo Case', *The Furrow*, 59 (February 2008), pp. 67–76.
Hamel, Ronald P., and James J. Walter (eds), *Artificial Nutrition and Hydration and the Permanently Unconscious Patient: The Catholic Debate*, Georgetown University Press, 2007.
Walter, James J., and Thomas A. Shannon (eds), *Contemporary Issues in Bioethics: A Catholic Perspective*, Rowman & Littlefield, 2005, part four.

NOTES

1. English Catholic Bishops, *The Tablet*, August 1993: 'There is a debate about whether it is correct to classify tube feeding as medical treatment. However the debate is resolved, it can be reasonable to stop tube feeding if a patient is in the final phase of dying or if the method of tube feeding involves excessive risks or burdens for a patient.'
2. The Irish Medical Council, for example, argued that 'access to nutrition and hydration is one of the basic needs of human beings. This remains so even when, from time to time, this need can only be fulfilled by means of long established methods such as naso gastric and gastrostomy tube feeding.'
3. 'Patients, competently diagnosed to be in a persistent vegetative state or in an irreversible coma, remain human persons. Nonetheless, those individuals are stricken with a lethal pathology which, without artificial nutrition and hydration, will lead to death.' *Medical Ethics: Source of Catholic Teachings*, Kevin O'Rourke and Philip Boyle (eds), Second Edition, Georgetown University Press, 1993, pp. 161–162.
4. National Conference of Catholic Bishops Committee on Pro-Life Activities, 'Nutrition and Hydration: Moral and Pastoral Reflections', *Origins*, 21.44 (19 April 1992), p. 705.
5. See, for example, the contrasting approaches and conclusions of Kevin Kelly, 'A Medical and Moral Dilemma', *Month*, 26 (April 1993), pp. 138–144; John M. Grondelski, 'Removal of Artificially Supplied Nutrition and Hydration: A Moral Analysis', *Irish Theological Quarterly*, 55 (1989), pp. 291–302; Anthony Fisher, 'On Not Starving the Unconscious', *New Blackfriars*, 74 (March 1993), pp. 130–145.
6. *Catechism of the Catholic Church*, paragraphs 2278–2279; *Evangelium vitae*, paragraph 65.
7. A similar point was later made by Pope John Paul II in 'Papal Address on Food and Water', *Ethics and Medics*, 29 (June 2004): 'In this sense, it must be noted that this term, even when confined to the clinical context, is certainly not the most felicitous when applied to human beings.'
8. 'Papal Address on Food and Water', *Ethics and Medics*, 29 (June 2004).
9. Ibid.
10. For example, Norman Ford, 'The Debate Goes On', *The Tablet*, 1 May 2004, p. 8; Thomas Shannon and James Walter, 'Assisted Nutrition and Hydration and the Catholic Tradition', *Theological Studies*, 66 (2005), pp. 651–662;

John J. Paris, et. al, '*Quaestio Disputata*: Did Pope John Paul II's Allocution on Life-Sustaining Treatments Revise Tradition?', *Theological Studies*, 67 (2006), pp. 163–174.
11. Catholic Bishops of Florida, 27 August 2003. This statement was published in *The Case of Terri Schiavo*, edited by Arthur L. Caplan, James J. McCartney and Dominic A. Sisti, Prometheus Books, 2006, pp. 94–95.
12. Ibid. Emphasis mine.
13. Ibid., pp. 96–97. This statement was given on 28 February 2005.
14. Congregation for the Doctrine of the Faith, *Responses to Certain Questions Concerning Artificial Nutrition and Hydration*: http://www.vatican.va/roman_curia/congregations/cfaith/documents/rc_con_cfaith_doc_20070801_risposte-usa_en.html.
15. Congregation for the Doctrine of the Faith, *Commentary*: www.vatican.va/roman_curia/congregations/cfaith/documents/rc_con_cfaith_doc_20070801_nota-commento_en.html.
16. Ibid.
17. Ibid.
18. Ibid.
19. Ibid.

Section Three
Catholic Moral Teaching and the Individual

6 The Nature and Role of Personal Conscience

IN THE FIRST CHAPTER WE EXAMINED THE SOURCES used by the Catholic Christian tradition in the process of moral reflection and moral decision-making. The second source of moral wisdom emphasised the importance of the living faith community. Christians belong to a community who have, over two thousand years, pondered on the moral implications of human behaviour in light of the Gospel. The Christian community is a community of moral conviction and the bearer of a moral tradition that it makes available to all. This chapter will examine the role of the individual within this living faith community. How does the individual relate to the moral convictions of the community that are articulated in Church teaching? What happens if the moral convictions of the individual, on a particular issue, do not harmonise with those of the community? What is the role of the individual's conscience within a community of faith and moral conviction?

Within the Catholic moral tradition the role of conscience has been addressed and clarified over the centuries. The *Catechism of the Catholic Church* provides us with a very clear definition of the nature and role of conscience:

> Conscience is a judgement of reason whereby the human person recognises the moral quality of a concrete act that he is going to perform, is in the process of performing, or has already completed.[1]

Furthermore, it asserts that 'in all he says and does, man is obliged to follow faithfully what he knows to be just and right.'[2]

Conscience is an essential dimension of our human makeup that both compels and enables us to reflect on our lives and actions and to arrive at practical judgements about the rightness or wrongness of those actions. Conscience calls us to live by these judgements in order that we may live authentically human lives. Conscience, then, requires and enables us to be responsible moral agents who take ownership of our decisions and actions.

The *Catechism* reminds us that conscientious activity demands a level of interiority that enables one to 'be sufficiently present to him/herself in order to hear the voice of his conscience.'[3] Conscientious reflection requires that we in some way 'step back' in order to reflect on our lives and the particular choices confronting us. From the perspective of the Christian family, as we will see later when we examine the steps involved in the formation of conscience, meditation and prayerful reflection on the Scriptures, are essential dimensions of conscientious reflection leading to decisions.

Despite the clarity of the definition of conscience provided by the *Catechism*, there is still often confusion as to the nature and role of conscience. There are two misunderstandings of conscience that are frequently voiced in public debate that will, paradoxically, help us to clarify the true nature and scope of conscience. The first misunderstanding is to reduce conscience to blind obedience to Church authority. In this scenario, Catholic Christians follow the teaching of the Church faithfully and uncritically without ever 'owning' the process and judgements of conscience. Rather than working out of *conviction*, individual Catholics simply *conform* to the insights of a higher authority. The second misunderstanding is to reduce conscientious activity to something trivial, solitary and purely subjective. Conscientious activity, in this scenario, is synonymous with doing what you like without any serious reflection or engagement with others. In this understanding, personal freedom is exalted and becomes an end in itself. It is detached from the community dimension of our existence and from objective truth; freedom *for* the truth is replaced by freedom *from* the truth.[4]

Both of these understandings are inadequate and severely misrepresent what Church teaching and theological reflection have articulated about the nature and function of conscience. They are, indeed, a caricature of the tradition's understanding. Properly understood the Catholic tradition identifies two essential dimensions of conscience that need to be kept in creative tension. The first dimension recognises that we are each obliged to seek moral and religious truth and to live by that truth. The second dimension recognises that the education of our conscience is a lifelong task that involves, for the person of faith, a sincere dialogue with the richness of the Christian heritage.

The first aspect of conscience acknowledges that the search for truth is an essential and inescapable part of being human. Because of this we can rightly speak of conscience as sacred and privileged: 'Their conscience is people's most secret core and their sanctuary. There they are alone with God whose voice echoes in their depths.'[5] Through conscientious activity we each search for the truth and embrace that truth when we have found it. In this way we are enabled to live lives that are authentic, fully human and full of integrity.

> Deep within their consciences men and women discover a law which they have not laid upon themselves and which they must obey. Their dignity rests in observing this law, and by it they will be judged.[6]

And:

> A human being must always obey the certain judgement of his conscience. If he were deliberately to act against it, he would condemn himself.[7]

The search for truth, however, must be conducted in a way that is in harmony with our dignity as persons, that is, in the context of freedom. The Church and most civil societies assert that we have a fundamental human right to freely search for the truth about life and God and to freely embrace that truth.[8] It is 'however only in freedom that people can turn themselves towards what is good.'[9]

> All are bound to follow their conscience faithfully in every sphere of activity so that they may come to God, who is their last end. Therefore the individual must not be forced to act against conscience nor be prevented from acting according to conscience, especially in religious matters.[10]

The tradition also recognises that persons can make mistakes in their judgements of conscience. Because we are fallible and sinful human beings, we can err in our judgements about what is correct behaviour in a particular instance. The tradition called this the *erroneous conscience*. If a person genuinely strives to seek the truth through prayer, reflection and dialogue with others and still arrives at a moral conclusion that is objectively not in keeping with God's law, we describe their situation as one of 'invincible ignorance'. In such a scenario 'conscience goes astray through ignorance which it is unable to avoid, without thereby losing its dignity'.[11]

In this case, the dignity of the individual's conscience and conscientious decision is affirmed and they are not held to be morally responsible for their erroneous moral judgements. *Culpable ignorance*, on the other hand, applies in cases where the person at the centre of the moral dilemma 'takes little trouble to find out what is true and good or when conscience is by degrees almost blinded through the habit of committing sin'.[12] In these circumstances, the person, in effect, abandons the search for truth in favour of their own uncritical judgement and are judged to be morally responsible for the errors of their ways.

In summary, then, this first aspect of conscience recognises that each person is endowed with the capacity to reflect on life and on their behaviour in order that they may 'do what is good and to avoid evil'.[13] Every person is obliged to follow the dictates of their conscience in the search for what is good and in conformity with God's ways. The special role and sacredness we ascribe to conscience and conscientious activity, seen in the use of terms like 'sanctuary'[14] to describe conscience, is often called the 'primacy of conscience'. This can be seen, also, in the special honour or esteem in which we hold conscientious objectors today.

The search for truth or the good must, moreover, be conducted in freedom since freedom is an essential demand of human dignity. This freedom to search for, and embrace, religious and moral truth must be acknowledged and facilitated by society. Because of our fallibility and sinfulness, individuals can err in the process and conclusions of conscientious decision-making. However, the erroneous conscience retains its dignity once the person sincerely engages with the process of truth-finding.

The second dimension of conscience highlighted in the Catholic moral tradition is the obligation to inform and educate one's conscience by engaging with the life and wisdom of the faith community. This second claim flows naturally from our self-understanding as members of a community of faith. The Christian person is always understood as a person-in-community rather than as an isolated and detached individual. As such we exist as part of a family gathered around the person of Christ and the call of the Gospel. As people of faith we strive to respond to that call in our daily lives by allowing the person of Christ to give shape and direction to our actions, attitudes and imaginations. The Christian community, guided by the ongoing presence and gifts of the Holy Spirit, has reflected on human existence and on the significance of human actions for over two thousand years. It has, or, more accurately, is a font of wisdom that we should seriously engage with as we strive to determine the call of truth in our own lives and circumstances. This wisdom, as discussed in chapter one, is found in the living tradition of the Church, including, amongst other elements, the witness of holy men and women and the teaching of the Magisterium.

The tradition recognises that the education of conscience is an ongoing and, indeed, 'a lifelong task'.[15] Our moral sensitivity can be sharpened and our commitment to the call of the Gospel strengthened as we continue to pray and dialogue with others and, especially, those within the community of faith.

The *Catechism of the Catholic Church* provides a very rich list of elements that contribute to the education or formation of our consciences:

In the formation of conscience the Word of God is the light for our path, we must assimilate it in faith and prayer and put it into practice. We must also examine our conscience before the Lord's Cross. We are assisted by the gifts of the Holy Spirit, aided by the witness or advice of others and guided by the authoritative teaching of the Church.[16]

Several aspects of this text are deserving of further reflection. The first thing to be noted is the richness and variety of formative sources listed: Scripture, prayer, meditation, the gifts of the Holy Spirit, the witness and advice of other people and the teaching of the Church. The rich tapestry of the Christian life is identified and promoted as a source of nourishment and enlightenment for the process of conscience formation. Church teaching, though very important, is but one element within this rich heritage of Christian sources.

It is also noteworthy that Scripture and prayer are assigned a central role in the process of informing one's conscience. This serves as a timely reminder that conscience formation and conscientious reflection, leading to conscientious activity, are, for the person of faith, conducted in the context of prayer. The gifts of the Holy Spirit are also explicitly mentioned in the text from the *Catechism*. This is a powerful reminder of the presence of the Holy Spirit in our world and of the gifted nature of all believers. Through our participation in the life of the faith community and through our reception of the sacraments of Baptism and Confirmation, we are each given the gifts of the Holy Spirit. These gifts include those of wisdom, discernment and prudence. By opening ourselves to the Holy Spirit we can wisely discern God's ways, even in the most complex circumstances. The living presence of the

Holy Spirit within individuals and the community reminds us that discernment is a *gift* and *task* of the whole faith community and not just of the Magisterium. This truth was powerfully reflected in the *consultative* methodology employed by the American Catholic bishops in writing their pastoral letters on war and the economy.

The importance of the advice and wisdom of others in our search for the good is also clearly acknowledged in the text. This reminds us that the search for what is moral and good is a universal search, in which those around us also participate and which generates a source of moral wisdom. Those around us who reflect on their life experiences through the prism of their Christian faith provide us with a ready source of Christian insight.

Finally, the teaching of the Church is presented as an essential element in the formation of conscience. It is worth noting at the outset that the verb used, 'guided', is quite a gentle one that allows space for individual conscientious discernment. Because the role of Church teaching in the education of conscience is often highlighted and, quite frequently, misunderstood, I will briefly outline the content and limits of this role.

The duty to inform and educate our consciences within the faith community is clearly articulated in Church documents over the centuries: 'However, in forming their consciences the faithful must pay careful attention to the holy and certain teachings of the Church.'[17] This obligation to engage with the teaching of the Church was articulated more forcefully in another document of the Second Vatican Council:

> [T]he faithful, for their part, are obliged to submit to their bishop's decision, made in the name of Christ, in matters of faith and morals, and to adhere to it with a ready and respectful allegiance of mind.[18]

These texts from Vatican II and the text from the *Catechism* use different terms to describe the stance of the individual towards Church teaching. These terms do not, at first sight, sit too easily with one another: 'pay careful attention to', 'submit to their bishop's decision in matters of faith and morals' and 'are guided by the authoritative teaching of the Church'. In light of this apparent tension, it is important to tease out what the stance of the individual should be when approaching the teaching of the Church on a particular subject.

The attitude of the person of faith towards Church teaching should be, in the first place, one of reverence and respect. This is because the Church is the Church of Christ and is guided by the Holy Spirit as it journeys through different times, cultures and contexts. The Church is not on its own as it tries to discern the implications of the 'Good News' in a dynamic world. As a community alive with God's guiding presence it believes that it enjoys the charism of infallibility that 'extends to all those elements of doctrine, including morals, without which the saving truths of the faith cannot be preserved, explained, or observed'.[19]

This charism of infallibility, because it concerns itself with what is at the core of Christian faith and identity, has a limited relevance for those moral teachings that engages with specific complex issues.[20] For the person of faith, Church teaching is experienced and appreciated as a special source of wisdom. It is recognised as the fruit of prayerful deliberation by those in ministries of discernment and leadership in the Church. Such teaching should be engaged with an attitude of reverence and with a presumption about its truthfulness and adequacy. Family and friends presume, unless painful experience has taught them otherwise, that what their fellow family members tell them is truthful, directed towards their well-being and motivated by love. A similar presumption should inform the person of faith as he/she approaches the moral reflections and teachings of the Church.

Since most Church teaching in the area of morality falls outside the category of infallible teaching, believers must distinguish, as the Church herself does, between the different kinds of Church teaching and the differing levels of authority and certitude to be found there.[21] The American Catholic bishops, in their very significant pastoral letter on the morality of nuclear weapons and nuclear conflict,[22] clearly articulated this point: 'Indeed we stress here at the very beginning that not every statement in this letter has the same moral authority.'[23]

The bishops went on to identify the different kinds of teaching and the levels of authority and certitude associated with them:

> At times we reassert universally binding moral principles (e.g., non-combatant immunity and proportionality). At still other times we reaffirm statements of recent popes and the teaching of Vatican II. Again, at other times we apply moral principles to specific cases.[24]

In applying moral principles to specific cases, the bishops note:

> [P]rudential judgements are involved based on specific circumstances which can change or which can be interpreted differently by people of good will (e.g., the treatment of 'no first use'). However, the moral judgements that we make in specific cases, while not binding in conscience, are to be given serious attention and consideration by Catholics as they determine whether their moral judgements are consistent with the Gospel.[25]

More recently, the Pontifical Council for Justice and Peace affirmed that the Church's social doctrine is authentic Magisterium, which obligates Catholics, but acknowledged the following:

> The doctrinal weight of the different teachings and the assent required are determined by the nature of the particular teachings, by their level of independence from contingent and variable elements, and by the frequency with which they are invoked.[26]

These texts, and the theological tradition underpinning them, give us several overlapping criteria to assess the 'weight' of Church teaching. These criteria include the *nature* (encyclical letter, pastoral letter, homily), the *source* (the Pope, Ecumenical Council, National Bishops' Conference, individual bishops), the *type* (the identification of fundamental principles and values or the application of same to a specific context) and the *frequency* of the Church teaching.

Two examples that focus on the *type* of teaching may help to clarify the importance of these distinctions. Respect for human life and the dignity of the person are, for example, central to the moral message of Christianity. They are non-negotiable principles that help define the ethos of the Christian family and its engagement with society. It is not self-evident, however, how these universally binding principles can be respected in a particular set of circumstances. Differences arise, for example, as to how these values are best protected and honoured in the context of conflict and warfare. Does the embracing of these core principles lead inevitably to pacifism and to the rejection of all killing? Or does their acceptance allow for a qualified acceptance of killing under strict conditions like those contained in the 'just war doctrine'? An acceptance of the latter position could still lead to disagreement amongst conscientious people as to the morality of a specific war, for example, the war in Iraq, or specific strategies and weapons within war, for example, the possession or use of nuclear weapons. Decisions on these specific moral issues demand prudential judgements based on an assessment of all the facts available, and people of good will may disagree in how they assess the relevant information. A consequence of this reality is that within the Catholic moral tradition there are pacifists and advocates of the 'just war doctrine', those who judge the possession or use of nuclear weapons to be morally unacceptable and those who give them a qualified moral approval, and Catholics amongst those who support and oppose the death penalty.

Likewise, the principle of the universal destination of the world's goods and the principle of justice are central and non-negotiable elements of the Christian community's moral tradition. They are, like the previous example, at the heart of Christian identity. People may disagree, based on their prudential judgement of all the circumstances, on how these core principles are honoured in the social and economic spheres. Does the principle of justice, for example, demand the introduction of higher taxes and greater state intervention or commitment to a particular political philosophy? Decisions on these matters involve prudential judgements based on the information available. People may differ in their conscientious assessment of the available data and, thereby, reach different moral conclusions.[27] These two examples reveal that the application of fundamental values to concrete and complex circumstances can be open to a range of conscientious conclusions.

In summary, then, this second aspect of conscience, the need to adequately inform our conscience, reminds us of our nature as sons and daughters of God created in God's image. We are reminded that moral wisdom is available to us through prayerful reflection on the Scriptures, through our availing of the fruits of the Holy Spirit and through engaging with the wisdom and teaching of the community of faith that we belong to. As sons and daughters of God, we can avail of divine assistance in our conscientious search for what is right by engaging with the rich living tradition of the Christian family. This dimension of conscience serves as a powerful critique of individualism and subjectivism. We are not adrift in the world but connected to others through faith, family and love. Because of this it is both prudent and necessary to engage with others when making moral decisions. We should approach Church teaching with reverence and respect and see it as a privileged source of moral wisdom. However, in engaging with such teaching we must distinguish between the various kinds of Church teaching and the different levels of authority and certitude that accompany them.

The two aspects of conscience identified in this chapter – on the one hand, the sacred and obliging nature of conscience and, on the other hand, the obligation to adequately educate our consciences through prayer, reflection, dialogue with others and engagement with Church teaching – must be kept in a healthy creative tension. By collapsing the tension in favour of blind obedience to the voices of others or rugged individualism, we distort the role of conscience and, thereby, impede conscientious living.

Discussion Questions

1. 'It is important for every person to be sufficiently present to him/herself in order to hear and follow the voice of conscience' (*Catechism of the Catholic Church*, 1779). Why is this requirement of interiority important?

2. What are the most important elements to be considered in the 'formation' of conscience?
3. Is the role of the Holy Spirit in the process of moral discernment adequately appreciated?
4. Why should Church teaching be appreciated as a privileged source of moral guidance?

FURTHER READING

Bretzke, James T., *A Morally Complex World: Engaging Contemporary Moral Theology*, Liturgical Press, 2004, chapter 4.

Catechism of the Catholic Church, Veritas, 1994, paragraphs 1776–1802.

Curran, Charles E. (ed.), *Conscience: Readings in Moral Theology*, No. 14, Paulist Press, 2004.

John Paul II, Pope, *Veritatis splendor*, Veritas, 1993, paragraphs 54–64.

McNamara, Vincent, *The Call to be Human*, Veritas, 2010, chapter 14.

NOTES

1. *Catechism of the Catholic Church*, paragraph 1778.
2. Ibid.
3. Ibid., paragraph 1779.
4. For a critique of this caricature of conscience see Pope John Paul II's, *Veritatis splendor*, Veritas, 1993, paragraphs 54–64.
5. *Constitution on the Church in the Modern World*, paragraph 16.
6. Ibid., paragraph 16.
7. *Catechism of the Catholic Church*, paragraph 1790.
8. 'No authentic progress is possible without respect for the natural and fundamental right to know the truth and live according to that truth.' Pope John Paul II, *Centesimus annus*, Veritas, 1991, paragraph 29.
9. *Constitution on the Church in the Modern World*, paragraph 17.
10. *Declaration on Religious Freedom*, paragraph 3.

11. *Church in the Modern World*, paragraph 16.
12. Ibid.
13. Ibid.
14. Ibid.
15. *Catechism of the Catholic Church*, paragraph 1784.
16. Ibid., paragraph 1785.
17. *Declaration on Religious Freedom*, paragraph 14.
18. *Dogmatic Constitution on the Church*, paragraph 25.
19. *Catechism of the Catholic Church*, paragraph 2035.
20. The nature and scope of infallible teaching is set out in *Lumen gentium*, paragraph 25.
21. For a full treatment of this subject see Francis A. Sullivan, SJ, *Creative Fidelity: Weighing and Interpreting Documents of the Magisterium*, Gill & Macmillan, 1996.
22. American Catholic Bishops, *The Challenge of Peace: God's Promise and Our Response*, Incorporated Catholic Truth Society, 1983.
23. Ibid., paragraph 9. See also US Conference of Catholic Bishops, *Forming Consciences for Faithful Citizenship*, 2007, paragraph 33.
24. Ibid.
25. Ibid., paragraph 10.
26. Pontifical Council for Justice and Peace, *Compendium of the Social Doctrine of the Church*, Veritas, 2005, paragraph 80.
27. An example from Irish history may be instructive in terms of the criteria to be considered when evaluating the 'weight' of Church teaching. Bishop Cohalan of Cork, in a Pastoral Letter, excommunicated all those involved in the War of Independence based on his assessment of that conflict. No other Irish bishop followed his example. See Pádraig Corkery, 'Bishop Daniel Cohalan of Cork on Republican Resistance and Hunger Strikes', *Irish Theological Quarterly*, 67 (2002), pp. 113–124.

Section Four

Catholic Moral Teaching and Society

7 Morality and the Civil Law

IN THE PREVIOUS CHAPTERS I HAVE TRIED TO OUTLINE, in as succinct a way as possible, the stance of the Catholic moral tradition on certain contemporary bioethical issues. This overview of bioethics will be, I hope, informative and helpful for those within and outside the Catholic faith community who are interested in or deeply involved with some of these contemporary issues.

This last chapter will attempt to look at the bigger picture by moving from the beliefs of a particular faith community to the content of civil legislation in society. How should the civil law be framed in a modern pluralistic society where people of different faiths, cultures and philosophical worldviews inhabit the same 'space'? What view of the world or understanding of morality should be reflected in what the civil law permits or prohibits? Is the opposition of the Catholic moral tradition to, for example, embryonic stem cell research a sufficient reason for the civil law to prohibit such research?

These are important questions that have been debated in the past and are the subject of ongoing debate in many societies. The Devlin-Hart debate in England, on the content of the civil law on prostitution and homosexual acts between consenting adults, is a standard reference point for this discussion and provides us with two very different approaches to the relationship between civil law and morality.[1] Lord Devlin, in brief, argued that every society is built on a shared morality and that the civil law has a legitimate interest in curtailing actions that conflict with that shared morality. This shared morality is, in his framework of understanding, the foundation stone on which society is built. All breaches of that morality are, in principle, of interest to the civil law because they could undermine this foundation and cause society to come tumbling down. Professor Hart, in contrast, assigned a more limited role to the civil law in society. He argued that the civil law has no interest in immorality *per se*, but has a legitimate interest in preventing those actions that cause harm to others. In the course of this debate between Lord Devlin and Professor Hart, the detail and nuances of both approaches were clearly identified.

The debate on the relationship between the civil law and morality has moved on since the Devlin-Hart debate both in terms of the intellectual frameworks proposed and the subjects considered. Today's debate on the content of the civil law centres on issues like euthanasia, the recognition of same sex marriages and the regulating of reproductive cloning. These issues are the subject of debate in society because, in the first place, people disagree on whether these actions are 'right', 'moral' or 'appropriate'. Secondly, people differ in their understanding of the purpose and goal of the civil law in a modern democracy. Should the civil law, when dealing with disputed moral issues, for example, reflect the views of the majority in society, those of the minority or some middle compromise position?

The relationship between morality and the civil law is a complex one. It is true to say, on the one hand, that there is a relationship between what the civil law permits or prohibits in society and what people judge to be right or wrong. The law prohibiting murder or stealing, for example, is enforceable in society because most people believe that these actions are morally unacceptable. On the other hand, the scope and content of morality is different from that of the civil law. Nobody would expect the civil law to prohibit all that they consider to be immoral. Indeed, there are areas of life that we consider to be none of the law's business. The civil law, moreover, is limited by what is practicable and enforceable. Morality and the content of the civil law, therefore, overlap but they are not identical. The civil law has a different goal to the goal of, say, a religiously motivated moral code. The goal of the latter could loosely be understood in terms of moral growth, spiritual maturity or holiness. The goal of the former could be formulated more modestly in terms of protecting the common good and creating the conditions that enable people to go about their lives in safety.

LAW AND MORALITY IN THE CATHOLIC MORAL TRADITION
The understanding of the relationship between the civil law and morality within the Catholic tradition was, over the ages, complicated and obscured by the relationship between the Church and the State. The history of the Church's relationship with the State, and the theology underpinning it, is complex and a detailed analysis of it is outside the parameters of this undertaking. It had a profound impact, however, on the understanding of the scope and content of the civil law that prevailed within Catholic theology up to the reforms of Vatican II.

The approach that held sway until Vatican II, in brief, began with the claim that everyone, including the State, has an obligation to serve God and objective truth. The State, in fulfilling this duty, could not treat truth and error or, indeed, all religions in the same way. 'Truth has rights, error has no rights' is a well-known catchphrase that succinctly sums up this approach. Working out of this framework of understanding, the State was obliged to promote and protect the truth and, when practicable, prohibit error. The key and obvious question that needs to be asked at this stage concerns the nature and content of truth. The response in Catholic theology to this question was clear and unambiguous: truth is located in the Catholic Church and her teachings. Therefore, the argument concluded, the State must promote and protect the Catholic Church and her teachings and, when practicable, prohibit what is contrary to Catholic teaching. This understanding of the relationship between Church and State, and its implications for the relationship between law and morality, prevailed in theology and in practice almost until Vatican II.

This mindset is seen most dramatically in the interventions of nineteenth-century popes and in the *Syllabus of Errors* of Pius IX.[2] The following propositions were amongst those *condemned* in the *Syllabus*:

> 15. Every man is free to embrace and to profess the religion he has judged by the light of reason to be true. ...
>
> 77. In our day, it is no longer advisable that the Catholic religion should be considered the only religion of the state, to the exclusion of all other forms of worship. ...
>
> 78. It is therefore quite right to make legal provision, as has been done in some Catholic countries, for foreigners going there to be able to engage in the public exercise of their particular forms of worship.

In effect, this theological framework, grounded in the *rights of truth*, meant that the Catholic tradition was religiously intolerant and insisted that, when possible, the civil law curtail the religious and moral freedoms of non-Catholics in society and prohibit actions that were contrary to the Catholic moral tradition.

The implications of this theological framework can be seen in the history of Church-State relations in Ireland prior to Vatican II. Though the Irish Constitution recognised and guaranteed religious freedom in Ireland, the content of civil legislation on disputed moral issues reflected the moral position of the majority Catholic tradition. This was an expectation of the Irish Catholic bishops and is clearly seen in their interventions in the area of civil legislation in the 1940s and 1950s. The bishops, for example, in 1950 and 1959, opposed the introduction of legislation permitting the opening of public houses on Sundays[3] and, between 1950 and 1953, opposed the Mother and Child Scheme of Dr Noel Browne. They opposed these pieces of legislation on the grounds that they were contrary to Catholic social and moral teaching on Sunday observance and the principle of subsidiarity. Implicit in their statements is the understanding that in a (Catholic) country like Ireland, the civil law should be in harmony with Catholic moral teaching.[4] It is important to point out that this understanding of the relationship between law and morality was accepted by the vast majority of Irish legislators during this time, as can be seen in the following piece of correspondence between the Taoiseach and the Minister for Health:

> I have no doubt that all my colleagues and, in particular, yourself would not be party to any proposals affecting moral questions which would or might come into conflict with the definite teaching of the Catholic Church.[5]

For a variety of reasons, including, no doubt, the intervention of the Irish bishops, these pieces of legislation were not immediately enacted. It is interesting to note that the second attempt to change the liquor laws with regard to Sunday trading, made in 1959, was again opposed by the bishops on the grounds that such legislation was contrary to the commandments and Catholic moral teaching. In this case, the legislators approved the legislation despite the intervention of the Irish bishops. This incident is probably indicative of a change in the mind of the legislator concerning the appropriate relationship between the Church and the State and between the civil law and morality. At this time also, theologians within the Catholic tradition were striving to construct a different theological framework that would enable a different understanding of the relationship between Church and State and, consequently, between the civil law and morality. Foremost amongst these theologians was the American Jesuit, John Courtney Murray. His scholarly work helped lay the foundation for the *Declaration on Religious Freedom* of Vatican II.[6]

THE DECLARATION ON RELIGIOUS FREEDOM

The *Declaration on Religious Freedom* engaged with the question of religious freedom in society and the relationship between Church and State from a very different perspective from that seen in earlier Church pronouncements. There is an acceptance in the document that the Church and the State have very different origins, competencies and goals. The Church's mission is to proclaim the truths of the Gospel and all it demands of the State is the freedom to pursue this mission. The document also recognises that the State is not competent in the area of religion and that its competencies and duties lie elsewhere. Significantly, the document placed the *rights of the person*, rather than the *rights of truth*, at its very centre. This is a very important shift in emphasis that has profound implications for how we understand religious and moral freedom in society.

The *foundations* and *content* of the right to religious freedom were elaborated in the opening paragraphs of the *Declaration*:

> The Vatican Council declares that the human person has a right to religious freedom. Freedom of this kind means that all people should be immune from coercion on the part of individuals, social groups and every human power so that, within due limits, nobody is forced to act against his convictions nor is anyone to be restrained from acting in accordance with his convictions in religious matters. … The Council further declares that the right to religious freedom is based on the very dignity of the human person as known through the revealed word of God and by reason itself. This right of the human person to religious freedom must be given such recognition in the constitutional order of society as will make it a civil right.[7]

Central to this affirmation of the right to religious freedom in society is an understanding that all persons are obliged and driven to search for the truth about life, God and existence. The right to religious freedom is not, therefore, founded on or encouraging of indifference to religious and moral truth. It insists, however, that the search for religious and moral truth must be conducted in a manner that is in keeping with the dignity of the human person, that is, in freedom:

> The search for truth, however, must be carried out in a manner that is appropriate to the dignity and social

nature of the human person: that is, by free enquiry with the help of teaching or instruction, communication and dialogue.[8]

The *Declaration* recognised that the search for religious and moral truth is a fundamental and essential aspect of the human condition. It argued that the State, in its service of the person and the human family, must honour this human dimension by recognising it as a civil right. Furthermore, it recognised that the facilitating of religious and moral freedom in society contributes to the common good of society because it enables authentic human living. Living out of personal conviction, rather than responding to coercion, enables the person to blossom and grow towards maturity.

The *Declaration* recognised that, like all other rights exercised in society, the right to religious and moral freedom may at times be curtailed by the State in its role as protector of the common good. It proposed two criteria to govern the limiting of religious freedom in society: *a moral limit* and a *legal limit*. The moral limit it proposed was that of the responsible use of freedom. This limit is, of course, self-imposed and self-regulated. Individuals should use their freedom in a way that is attentive to the rights and privileges of others in society. The legal limit proposed in the *Declaration*, to be used by the State to regulate freedom in society, is that of 'public order'.[9] The State should facilitate religious and moral freedom in society unless the exercise of this freedom undermines the public order of society. The content of public order was understood in the *Declaration* to have a three-fold content: *justice, public morality* and *peace*. Outside of this limit, the *Declaration* embraced the principle that 'the freedom of humankind be respected as far as possible, and curtailed only when and in so far as necessary'.[10]

The criterion of public order is a very useful one in helping society and individuals determine the level of religious and moral freedom that is acceptable in society. Though the constituent elements – justice, public morality, peace – need to be unpacked, they do provide objective, non-religious criteria that can facilitate a public debate on the content of the civil law on issues, like euthanasia, that are morally disputed.

We will now examine some post-Vatican II Church documents, from the universal and local Church, that utilise the insights and spirit of the *Declaration on Religious Freedom* when discussing the role of the civil law in society.

The Irish Catholic bishops, in a statement in 1973 concerning a proposal to legalise the sale of contraceptives, embraced the understanding of the relationship between law and morality articulated at Vatican II. For the first time they explicitly acknowledged that the civil law was not obliged to protect or promote Catholic morality *per se*.

> The question at issue is not whether artificial contraception is morally right or wrong. The clear teaching of the Catholic Church is that it is morally wrong. ... It does not follow, of course, that the State is bound to prohibit the importation and sale of contraceptives. There are many things which the Catholic Church holds to be morally wrong and no one has ever suggested, least of all the Church herself, that they should be prohibited by the State. ... What the legislators have to decide is whether a change in the law would, on balance, do more harm than good, by damaging the character of the society for which they are responsible.[11]

Subsequent statements from the Irish bishops, in the 1970s and 1980s, on the content of the civil law also recognised the distinction between the content of Catholic moral teaching and the role of the legislator.[12] In legislating for contraceptives, the legislator had many things to take into account, including: the importance of maximising the zone of moral and religious freedom in society; the rights of those who on religious or moral grounds disagree with Church teaching on the use of artificial contraceptives; the enforceability of a law prohibiting the sale of contraceptives; and the impact of the availability of artificial contraceptives on public morality. Having considered all these factors, the legislator had to make a prudential judgement about the kind of legislation that best served the rights of the person and the welfare of society.

On the global stage, *Donum vitae*, after clearly outlining the approach and conclusions of the Catholic moral tradition to developments in reproductive technology, dedicated its last chapter to the relationship between morality and the civil law. It began its reflection by defining the task of the civil law as follows: [T]o ensure the common good of people through the recognition of and the defence of fundamental rights and through the promotion of peace and of public morality.'[13]

With regard to fundamental rights, it specifically identified every human being's right to life and physical integrity from the moment of conception until death. On the basis of this understanding of the role of the civil law and of fundamental rights, it urged legislators to prohibit IVF and other procedures that result in the destruction or manipulation of the embryo.

Several years later, *Evangelium vitae* addressed the issue in similar terms; the duty of the legislator and civil law is to protect fundamental rights, peace and public morality.[14] It argued that first among these fundamental rights is 'the inviolable right to life of every innocent human being.'[15] On the basis of this understanding, it concluded that 'a civil law authorising abortion or euthanasia ceases by that very fact to be a true, morally binding civil law'.[16] In its treatment of the nature and value of democracy, it contended that the moral value of democracy is not automatic but depends, rather, on the 'morality of the ends which it pursues and of the means which it employs'.[17] The basis of an acceptable democracy is one where its values are based on 'an objective moral law which, as the "natural law" written in the human heart, is the obligatory point of reference for civil law itself'.[18]

To enable human flourishing and the protection of human dignity, the civil law must be founded on what is objective, rather than on that which is provisional or changeable. Since the civil law and the political system are at the service of the human person, they must be rooted in a proper understanding of the nature and dignity of the person.[19] Consequently, *Evangelium vitae* argues, democratic governments should encourage and facilitate debate about the nature of human dignity and objective morality, rather than encouraging ethical relativism or moral scepticism. People should be encouraged to work together to understand better the nature of the human person and the fundamental rights that belong to the person, since these are the foundations on which society and the law must be constructed if they are to endure.

There are several important points to be noted in this limited sample of references, from the universal and local church to the role of the civil law in society: there is a clear recognition that the role and scope of the civil law and the moral law are different; the right to religious and moral freedom in society is affirmed as a fundamental human right rooted in the dignity of the person; democracy and the civil law are understood to be at the service of the human person and community; the exercise of freedom in society can be curtailed when it infringes on fundamental human rights, disturbs the peace of society or undermines the public morality of society.

The framework for understanding the scope of religious and moral freedom in society, evident in these statements and built on the insights of the *Declaration on Religious Freedom*, has consequences for the tone and shape of the Church's contribution to the societal debate on the content of civil legislation. It enables the Church to voice its opposition to a particular freedom in society, not on the basis of Catholic moral teaching *per se*, but on the basis of that freedom's opposition to the public order of society. The Church does not demand that the State respect Catholic moral teaching *per se* in its legislation, but rather that it protects fundamental human rights and the dignity of the person. So, for example, the Church continues to campaign against the legalisation of embryo destruction not because it is contrary to Catholic teaching, but because it is contrary to the principle of justice and respect for human life. This enables the Church to enter into the public square and debate the merits of legislation using language and principles – justice, public morality, fundamental rights, public order – that have a universal acceptance.

The general framework proposed here – that the civil law in its service of the person should recognise and protect fundamental rights – is one that is supported by most people. Most people would also accept that the civil law and the foundations of society should be built on what is objective and true, rather than on ideas that are provisional, changeable or false. Difficulty arises, however, when we try to 'unpack' what these terms mean. People of good will may disagree in their understanding of the terms 'fundamental rights' , 'justice' or 'objective morality'. There is, for example, an energetic debate about the identification and ordering of fundamental rights and the resolution of conflicting rights.

The framework for understanding the relationship between morality and the civil law outlined in Church documents give us criteria that are useful but, for the reasons cited above, do not readily lead to agreement in society on the content of the civil law. Consequently, a feature of many modern pluralistic democracies is that reasonable people, motivated by the best intentions, disagree when legislating for specific issues. Given this context, the Christian community has a very important role to play in the discussion and debate that surrounds the enacting of legislation on sensitive moral issues. As a community of faith and the bearer of a moral tradition, it is obliged to make its contribution based on its understanding of the issues involved. Its contribution to the debate must always, of course, be in harmony with the spirit and content of the Gospel: respectful, honest and generous. It must strive to articulate clearly how a proposed piece of legislation would infringe on fundamental human rights, societal peace or public morality. In doing this it must draw upon empirical data and human experience, rather than specifically Christian sources. The contribution of the Catholic community should be robust but delivered in a manner that is respectful of the distinction between the roles of the civil and moral law. Equally, it should be appreciative of the value of religious and moral freedom in society and the contribution that such freedom makes to the common good. It should, moreover, be delivered in a spirit that recognises and respects the deeply held religious and moral convictions of others and their right to live by those convictions in society. Finally, the starting point of any contribution from the Catholic tradition should include an embracing of the spirit and content of the

Declaration on Religious Freedom on the scope of religious and moral freedom in society. The presumption is in favour of religious and moral freedom in society. Those who want to limit freedom must prove their case by appealing to the public order of society.

DISCUSSION QUESTIONS
1. What are the roots and content of the right to religious freedom in society as set out in the *Declaration on Religious Freedom*?
2. 'But the value of democracy stands or falls with the values which it embodies and promotes' (*Evangelium vitae*, 70). What are the values that should underpin democracy?
3. 'Certainly the purpose of civil law is different and more limited in scope than that of the moral law' (*Evangelium vitae*, 71). What is the role of the civil law in a modern pluralist democracy?
4. On what grounds should the Catholic Church in Ireland frame a response to legislative proposals on reproductive technologies, embryonic stem cell research and euthanasia?

FURTHER READING
Congregation for the Doctrine of the Faith, *Donum vitae*, Part III.
---, *Doctrinal Note on Some Questions Regarding the Participation of Catholics in Political Life*, Veritas, 2002.
John Paul II, Pope, *Evangelium vitae*, paragraphs 68–75.
United States Conference of Catholic Bishops, *Readings on Catholics in Political Life*, Washington, DC, 2006.

NOTES
1. Patrick Devlin, *The Enforcement of Morals*, Oxford University Press, 1965; H.L. Hart, *Law, Liberty and Morality*, Oxford University Press, 1963.

2. Pope Pius IX, *Syllabus of Errors*, 1864. See J. Neuner and J. Dupuis, *The Christian Faith*, revised edition, Christian Classics, 1975, pp. 269–271.
3. 'Statement on Liquor Law', *The Furrow*, 1 (1950), pp. 363–366; 'Statement on Liquor Law', *Irish Ecclesiastical Record*, 92 (1959), pp. 129–130.
4. For an account of this period in Irish history, see John H. Whyte, *Church and State in Modern Ireland 1923–79*, Second Edition, Gill & Macmillan, 1980, chapters 7 and 8. The complete correspondence between the Irish bishops and the Irish Government on the Mother and Child Scheme are reproduced in Appendix B.
5. Ibid., p. 429.
6. John Courtney Murray, *The Problem of Religious Freedom*, Newman Press, Maryland, 1965; John Courtney Murray (ed.), *Religious Liberty: An End and a Beginning*, MacMillan, New York, 1966.
7. *Declaration on Religious Freedom*, paragraph 2.
8. Ibid., paragraph 3.
9. Ibid., paragraph 7.
10. Ibid.
11. Irish Catholic Bishops' Conference, 'Statement on Legislation for Contraceptives', *L'Osservatore Romano*, 13 December 1973, p. 12.
12. For example, Irish Catholic Bishops' Conference, 'Public Morality', *The Furrow*, 27 (1976), pp. 444–445; 'Proposed Legislation on Family Planning and Contraception', *The Furrow*, 29 (1978), pp. 525–527; 'Health (Family Planning) Act 1979', *Irish Times*, 29 October 1980, p. 5.
13. *Donum vitae*, Section III.
14. *Evangelium vitae*, paragraph 71.
15. Ibid.
16. Ibid., paragraph 72.
17. Ibid.
18. Ibid., paragraph 70.
19. See also Congregation for the Doctrine of the Faith, *Doctrinal Note on Some Questions Regarding the Participation of Catholics in Political Life*, 2002, www.vatican.va/roman_curia/congregations/cfaith/documents/rc_con_cfaith _doc_20021124_politica_en.html, paragraph 3: 'The Church recognises that while democracy is the best expression of the direct participation of citizens in political choices, it succeeds only to the extent that it is based on a correct understanding of the human person.'